The Weight Of Expectations: A Doctor's Fall

Sibongiseni Masengemu

Published by Sibongiseni Masengemu, 2025.

THE WEIGHT OF EXPECTATIONS: A DOCTOR'S FALL

First edition. December 4, 2025.

ISBN: 979-8232425753

Written by Sibongiseni Masengemu.

Table of Contents

The Weight of Expectations: A Doctor's Fall

Chapter 1: The Burden of Success

Dr. Thabo Mthembu was not just a man; he was a monument. His success, bought with endless late nights under the cold, fluorescent hospital lights, belonged not just to him but to every proud, struggling soul in the sprawling township of KwaMashu. When he pulled his first German sedan into his mother's dusty yard—a gleaming black shape alien to the noise and close-packed homes—it was a communal triumph, a validation of collective hope. This collective ownership, however, came with a crushing tariff: the need for constant, tangible proof that he was still ascending.

His life, once driven by the simple goal of healing, became dictated by the relentless demands of his public image, physically embodied by his three wives. **Nomusa**, his first wife, was the anchor to tradition, settled in a sturdy, functional house near the city center. She was quiet, her needs communicated through persistent, unspoken expectation: sponsoring a nephew's education, paying the higher *lobola* for a relative, maintaining the respectful distance expected of a senior wife. She represented his history, and her validation was his roots.

Zandile, the second, was the face of modernity. She demanded the suburban house, the international school fees, the tasteful art, and the specific brand of respect afforded to a doctor's wife in a new, aspirationally middle-class environment. She read home decor magazines and spoke of "networking" at the private schools. **Ayanda**, the youngest, was pure, costly vanity—diamonds for anniversaries, spontaneous trips to Cape Town he couldn't afford, and a constant thirst for validation that mirrored Thabo's own professional anxiety.

To maintain this trident of expectation required three parallel realities, three vastly different budgets, and three sets of emotional energy he no longer possessed.

The provincial hospital, for all its sterile efficiency, was a pressure cooker of professional status. Thabo earned well, but his colleagues, especially the senior specialists, spoke casually of offshore accounts, wine estates, and second passports. Thabo felt perpetually inadequate, a wealthy man in debt. When Dr. Van Zyl purchased a new, dark grey S-Class, Thabo's heart hammered not with mere envy, but with cold, financial panic. He *had* to upgrade his own sedan, even though his current vehicle was barely two years old.

The sales manager, seeing the desperate fatigue behind the doctor's eyes, cheerfully guided him through the paperwork for a devastating vehicle finance loan. "It's not just a car, Doctor," the manager had purred, "it's your mobile office. Your image. Your worth. Patients trust success." Thabo signed, believing the lie, linking his professional competence to the thickness of his car's leather seats.

The true abyss, however, was the house. Zandile's relentless, whispered campaign had worn him down. The move to the suburbs—a place of manicured lawns, high security, and overwhelming silence—was the point of no return. It was a palace of glass and exposed brick, a four-bedroom monolith that whispered of arrival.

He signed the bond papers in a rush, a tremor running through his hand that no amount of medical training could suppress. The repayment: R38,000 per month. His net salary was R45,000. He had factored in "future bonuses" and "private consultation fees" that existed only in his mind. The reality was a gaping, immediate, non-negotiable deficit. The electric fence was installed not to keep intruders out, but to lock him in with the impossible debt.

The first month in the new house felt like occupying a tomb. He walked through the cavernous living room, the imported leather sofa cool and resistant beneath his touch. He was surrounded by space, silence, and the profound, isolating knowledge that he was deeply, permanently insolvent. His bank account was a flatlining trace, and his entire existence was leveraged against a crumbling facade.

The phone notification arrived one evening like a death knell: a final demand for the loan taken to buy Ayanda's bespoke walk-in closet furniture. The interest rate felt predatory, the balance insurmountable. Thabo stared at the screen, the blue light reflecting in his pupils. His medical degree, his three wives, his three houses—they were not symbols of success. They were chains, and Dr. Thabo Mthembu, the proud son of the *kasi*, was officially drowning in the clean, silent waters of the suburban dream. He had bought a life that required him to perpetually be someone he was not. The only solution, he realized with a sick lurch, was not to earn more, but to find a different kind of currency.

Chapter 2: The Whispers of a Shortcut

The sterile efficiency of the provincial hospital was the only place Thabo felt partially anchored, but even that sanity was slipping. The financial noose tightened daily, transforming professional interactions into gauntlets of potential humiliation. He began avoiding the staff canteen, feigning hurriedness to escape the indignity of petty costs. The inevitable finally happened one afternoon. His credit card was declined for a simple R50 coffee purchase from the mobile vendor—in front of three junior nurses he was supposed to be mentoring. The small, buzzing sound of the rejected transaction felt louder than a gunshot. Thabo's face burned with a shame that was corrosive, a public stripping of the respect he had spent two decades earning.

That night, alone in the echoing suburban house—Zandile and the children were mercifully visiting family—Thabo didn't seek comfort. He dialed Sipho, his old schoolmate, a man who had left the path of conventional employment early and emerged years later driving cars Thabo could only dream of, with a fortune made in opaque "logistics and distribution."

They met downtown, in a club layered with history and thick cigar smoke, far from both the sterile hospital and the silent suburbs. Sipho greeted him with an unnervingly accurate assessment.

"You look like death, Doc," Sipho boomed, waving away the waiter as Thabo fumbled for his wallet. "My treat. Put that away. You can't afford to look like a beggar when you are meant to be a king."

Thabo laid out his predicament, meticulously detailing the debt, the pressure from his wives, the sheer exhaustion of maintaining the lie. He spoke of interest rates and bond repayments, hoping for a business solution, perhaps a high-interest loan.

Sipho didn't offer sympathy or a loan. He leaned back, exhaling a plume of cigar smoke that made Thabo wince and tear up slightly. "You're thinking like a doctor, Thabo. Logic, systems, bank statements. The white man's way. The truth is, the world isn't logical. It needs to be persuaded by something stronger than paper."

"I don't understand," Thabo repeated, his throat dry.

Sipho smiled, a knowing, weary smile that didn't reach his eyes. "That world you bought—the suburbs, the degrees, the bond—it's built on paper and interest. But real power, lasting prosperity, comes from grounding yourself in something older. Something hungry. You need *isidliso*, my friend. The spiritual transaction."

Thabo felt a cold knot of dread tighten in his stomach. He knew the word. It referred to dark practices, to using forces best left alone to guarantee unnatural prosperity. It was the stuff of whispers, fear, and profound cultural taboos—an inversion of the healer's path.

"It's not what you think," Sipho rushed to reassure him, sensing the panic. "No curses, no direct harm to people. The snakes, the rats, the pots... they are simply conduits. Vessels. They attract fortune. Think of them as a very hungry, very efficient investment portfolio. You feed them, and they feed your wealth. They multiply the cash you put into the system."

Sipho explained the rules with chilling calmness. The "investment tools" would require privacy—a locked room or shed. Their existence must be an absolute secret, especially from his wives, whose feminine energy might interfere. And their nourishment had to be continuous and unique, the kind of offerings that appeased powerful, demanding spirits.

"It costs money, yes, but it's an investment that pays in millions, not rands," Sipho urged, his eyes gleaming with the manic certainty of a successful fraudster. "You need to reset your luck, Thabo. You've let the debt swallow your spirit. This will make you unsinkable. The fortune is out there, Thabo. You just need to show it a way in."

Thabo thought of the final demand notice. He thought of his professional humiliation. He thought of his children's future being foreclosed. The shame was a burning acid, and the rational world had failed him utterly. He was a doctor, a man of science, contemplating a partnership with black magic.

"How do I... arrange this transaction?" Thabo asked, his voice a ghost of a rasp. He had crossed a boundary, and the crossing felt sickeningly easy, as if he had merely stepped from one dark room to another. He rationalized it as just a cultural remedy for financial bad luck. He rationalized it as just a bigger, scarier, but necessary loan.

Sipho clapped him on the shoulder, the gesture feeling heavy and final. "I'll arrange the introduction to the *nyanga* by the end of the week, Doctor. You take the chance. It's not harm. It's just business."

Thabo drank the rest of his whisky, the taste metallic and foul, like something already dead. He was now officially in partnership with the darkness, hoping it would save him from the suburbs.

Chapter 3: The Secret in the Shed

The transaction was swift, conducted in the dead of night at the *nyanga's* small, windowless shop on the outskirts of the city. The *nyanga*, a skeletal woman with eyes that seemed to hold all the smoke and shadows of the city's underbelly, took the last of Thabo's available cash—a sum that emptied his savings account entirely. In return, he received his dreadful "investment": a heavy, sealed wooden box containing the rats, a tall, repurposed cabinet holding the snake (a large, sluggish python, sleek and unsettlingly still), and three clay pots, dark and oily, wrapped in specific strips of colored cloth.

The drive back to the suburbs was a descent into psychological horror. The back seat of his expensive, financed car smelled of earth, stale herbs, and something metallic and cold—a scent that seemed to cling to his conscience. He installed them in the large garden shed behind the suburban house, reinforcing the door and adding a heavy, conspicuous padlock. This shed, once meant for gardening tools he never bought, became his sanctuary of ruin, his black altar to greed.

The *nyanga*'s instructions were specific, delivered in a low, rapid tongue that brooked no argument. The rats needed to be fed every night, the snake once a week, and the pots required a daily libation poured directly from Thabo's hands. She stressed that the required sustenance was potent. It needed **life force**, something highly concentrated, forbidden, and drawn from the very lifeblood of the city's energy.

Thabo's medical training was useless, but his access was unparalleled. He began his second, secret life, a routine of profound ethical violation. At the provincial hospital, the boundary between ethical practice and moral degradation dissolved. Working late, claiming to be preparing complex patient reports for the CMO, he would linger near the lab and the biohazard stations.

He started skimming off highly concentrated fluids from regulated biological waste, packaging specimens destined for incineration, or taking small, excised tissue samples—materials that would never be missed in the hospital's vast bureaucracy, but which were strictly forbidden to leave the premises. He used his knowledge of antiseptic procedures to carefully extract and package his vile offerings, his hands moving with the horrific precision of a man performing a perversion of surgery.

Each small act of theft was a sickening violation. He, Dr. Mthembu, the healer, the man who had sworn the Hippocratic Oath, was stealing bio-matter from the very institution that had given him status. He was contaminating his hands and his soul with transgression.

He would stash the foul packages in a hidden compartment he hastily built into his leather briefcase, carrying his grotesque offerings from the antiseptic white world of the hospital to the quiet, judgmental darkness of his suburban shed.

The nightly ritual became his sole, paranoid focus. He would wait until the whole house—when Zandile and Ayanda were home—was completely asleep, slipping out in the oppressive quiet of the suburbs, the electric fence humming softly like a restless predator. He would unlock the shed. The rats would scratch and gnaw at their feast in the dark. The snake would stir, its coils thick and cold, a heavy, silent promise. The pots sat on the floor, dark and oily, seeming to watch him, silent and expectant.

Thabo kept the secret with maniacal intensity, fueled by guilt and desperation. When Zandile complained about the faint, earthy odor that occasionally drifted from the back of the yard, blaming mold or dead leaves, Thabo shouted her down—an unprecedented, paranoid outburst. He became withdrawn, spending his off-hours either staring at bank statements that refused to decrease or locked in the shed, tending to his malignant fortune.

He waited for the tide to turn. He waited for the millions Sipho promised. He waited for the *isidliso* to work its magic.

A month passed. The debt collectors called three times a day. Ayanda demanded a vacation to Zanzibar he couldn't afford. The bond payment was officially overdue. The darkness he had embraced had not brought wealth. It had only brought him closer to the pit, dragging his medical soul and his physical sanity down with it. He was a wealthy man in his mind, but his bank account showed nothing but ruin, and the only thing multiplying was his overwhelming sense of dread.

Chapter 4: The Final Descent

The inevitable arrived not with a spectacular bang, but with the cold, measured efficiency of a bureaucratic review. A sharp-eyed, meticulous lab technician, puzzled by repeated, minor discrepancies in the biohazard ledger and noticing the strange late-night movements of a senior doctor, had escalated her concerns to the hospital administration. There was no direct proof of Thabo's shed rituals, but the ensuing investigation quickly uncovered enough inconsistencies and profound procedural breaches—missing tissue samples, unauthorized access logs—to flag him as a major operational and ethical risk.

The Chief Medical Officer, a grim-faced woman named Dr. Molefe, who had once been Thabo's mentor and greatest champion, called him into her office. The room felt small, the air heavy with disappointment. She didn't accuse him of theft or dark practices; she simply detailed the sheer instability of his recent performance: the missed shifts, the dangerous sloppiness in record keeping, the pervasive, undeniable smell of stale alcohol on his breath in the mornings, and the sheer fatigue that made him a liability in surgery. His reputation, once the pride of the hospital, was now shredded beyond repair.

"Dr. Mthembu," she said, looking past him at the wall, her voice emotionless, "we are terminating your employment immediately, effective today. Your medical license has been suspended by the Health Council pending a full ethical review. The findings are too severe to ignore. Please clear out your locker by the end of the day. Security will escort you from the premises."

Thabo stumbled out, the antiseptic hospital air suddenly thick and suffocating, the fluorescent lights burning his eyes. The one anchor holding him to his respectable life was gone. He was not just broke; he was unemployable, a pariah stripped of his professional identity.

The collapse of his personal life was swift and merciless, a dramatic, separate set of catastrophes. As the bank initiated foreclosure on the suburban house and the repossession agents took the second German car (leaving him only the small, hidden run-around), his three wives arrived—not together, but in separate, furious waves, each visit a scene of devastating clarity.

Nomusa, the eldest, arrived first. She stood quietly amidst the packing boxes, her face etched with profound, quiet devastation. "You chased a ghost, Thabo," she said, her voice barely a whisper. "You wanted to be more than what God made you. You took us away from what was real for a house that was empty. There is nothing left for me here." She took her children and returned to the small house in the inner city, leaving behind only a small, worn Bible, a silent critique of his moral failures.

Ayanda wept hysterically, collapsing onto the leather sofa (which was soon to be repossessed). Her grief was loud, frantic, and entirely self-centered, not for him, but for the loss of the wealth and lifestyle he had promised. She left for her sister's place, taking every last expensive, unearned item of furniture from her separate apartment.

Zandile, the most pragmatic, arrived last, presenting him simply with divorce papers. Her eyes were empty, hollowed out by betrayal. "You are not the man I married," she stated, her voice chillingly devoid of emotion. "You are a stranger who smells of rot and fear. I want nothing from you but your signature."

Alone, stripped of his prestige, his family, and his career, Thabo retreated into the deserted suburban house. He couldn't face the judgment of the *kasi*. He hid, sleeping in sweatpants on the floor, watching the news reports of his professional disgrace on a small, old television he hadn't yet sold. His drinking became constant. The rats scratched. The snake lay still. The pots demanded their offering, and the debt continued to mount. The *isidliso* had only accelerated his ruin, demanding payment while delivering nothing.

One night, completely gone in a bottle of cheap liquor, the twisted, desperate voice of the *nyanga*'s promise returned: the fortune needed a catalyst. It needed a final, ultimate violation to turn the tide. In his drunken haze, Thabo saw the world not as patients and people, but as sources of raw, potent fuel for the dark forces he had unleashed.

He staggered out of the house, grabbed the keys to his last remaining car, and drove aimlessly toward the edges of the city, consumed by a drunken, suicidal rage. In his mind, he wasn't driving, he was hunting, trying to satisfy the terrible hunger he felt was radiating from his backyard shed.

The drive was blurred, reckless, and terrifyingly close to a final, tragic act that would fulfill the darkness's true requirements. But just as the moral compass of his former life—the Hippocratic Oath, the memory of his father's stoic face—flickered one last time, he slammed on the brakes, swerving onto a patch of overgrown grass.

He wept, burying his face in the steering wheel, the stench of stale alcohol and fear filling the car. He had become a monster trying to feed monsters. The millions never came. Only the ruin.

"I wish I didn't take it," he sobbed into the quiet night, the phrase a self-condemnation, a complete acceptance of his own damnation. "I wish I didn't take it."

Chapter 5: The Reckoning

The morning after the disastrous drive was a study in brutal, physical reality. Thabo woke up stiff, aching, and covered in dried sweat, the sun slicing through the dusty windshield of the small car. The panic was gone, replaced by a cold, metallic clarity. The debt hadn't evaporated. The shame was permanent. The foreclosure was hours away.

He stumbled back into the house, which now echoed with a crushing, final emptiness. He was a prisoner awaiting execution. The final eviction notice, stamped with the bank's logo, was taped to the expensive imported refrigerator. The illusion was over. There was only one final, terrible task left—the closing of the spiritual ledger.

He retrieved a heavy garden spade from the corner of the empty garage and walked to the shed. He yanked the heavy padlock off, the sound echoing too loudly in the otherwise silent suburban street. The smell that rushed out was overwhelming—a potent mixture of stale offering, decay, and the metallic tang of something deeply unnatural.

He switched on the single bare bulb inside. The rats, the wretched conduits of his greed, scurried and squeaked, scrambling for cover. The great python, a thick, coiling mass of muscle and cold skin, lay motionless in its wooden cabinet, its eyes dull and unblinking. The three dark pots sat on the floor, their promised fortune exposed as a cruel, expensive lie.

Thabo didn't hesitate. He swung the spade, its heavy metal blade impacting the first pot with a sickening *thud*. The clay exploded into sharp shards, scattering oily earth and colored cloth across the concrete floor. He repeated the action, destroying the other two. With a wild, desperate energy, he overturned the wooden rat box, letting the vermin scramble out into the overgrown flowerbeds, reclaiming their ordinary, non-magical existence. He unlatched the snake's cabinet and flung the door wide open. The python, sensing the radical change, slowly uncoiled and slithered out, ignoring Thabo completely, disappearing into the dense shrubbery under the deck of the greening swimming pool, a silent symbol of his released dark attachment.

Thabo stood amidst the physical wreckage of his folly, sweating, trembling, and utterly ruined. He had banished the dark instruments, but the core corruption—the moral disease he had contracted at the hospital, the desperate greed in his heart—remained rooted in his soul. The *isidliso* had been a mirror, forcing him to sacrifice his integrity for a void.

His hands, once revered for their skill and precision, now felt foreign, rough, tainted by the illicit fluids they had carried and the reckless wheel they had gripped. He walked out, locking the shed door for the very last time, leaving the spiritual ruin locked away, even as his material world evaporated around him.

He gathered a few necessities—his medical diploma (now a useless, rolled-up piece of parchment), his worn Bible (a token of the goodness he had lost), and the last bottle of liquor—and walked away from the house, leaving his keys on the pristine white counter, a final gesture of surrender. He didn't look back at the suburban mansion, the symbol of the life that had swallowed him whole. He was no longer Dr. Mthembu; he was just a ghost, walking back toward the anonymity of the city.

Chapter 6: The Silence

Months later, the house stood vacant, a monument to failed ambition. The bank had taken possession, the grass had yellowed, and the pool had turned a stagnant, toxic green. It was a casualty of the property boom, a foreclosure statistic, its brief moment as a gilded cage for Dr. Mthembu forgotten by the surrounding community.

Miles away, in the smoke-filled, mahogany-paneled club, Sipho leaned back on his expensive leather seat, reviewing his complex ledger of "investments." He heard a brief, cynical mention of Thabo's ruin through an associate—the loss of the house, the wives, the suspended license.

Sipho merely shrugged, lighting a freshly rolled cigar with a golden lighter. "He was weak," Sipho muttered. "The spirits demand conviction. He tried to buy power with a doctor's hesitation. It was a simple business transaction that went sour. Thabo's failure was his own moral failing, not mine." Sipho quickly forgot Thabo, moving on to the next desperate client looking for a shortcut to the riches they believed they deserved.

Meanwhile, Thabo Mthembu found himself precisely where he had sworn he would never be again: back in the deep anonymity of the urban sprawl, taking shelter in a cheap, shared room on the fringes of the *kasi* he had once ascended from. He was unrecognizable now. The tailored suits were replaced by ill-fitting, worn, and grease-stained clothing. The physician's dignity was gone, replaced by a haunted, perpetually weary look and a physical stoop.

He spent his days doing manual labor for cash at a distribution depot, scrubbing floors or clearing debris, tasks that demanded only physical exhaustion, leaving his mind mercifully numb. He avoided the main streets where he might be recognized, hiding his disgrace, afraid of the contempt of the very people he had once been meant to represent.

He was sober now, but the sobriety brought with it a crushing, inescapable awareness. The great life he sought—the status, the power, the visibility—had not been taken by the suburbs or the debt collectors. It had been systematically dismantled piece by piece by his own desperate, greedy choices, starting with the first moment he chose image over integrity.

He paused his work one afternoon, wiping sweat and dust from his brow. He stared at his hands. They were rough, scarred, and strong, no longer the clean, educated hands of a surgeon, but the hands of a working man.

He remembered the final, terrified instant in the car, the moral abyss he had stared into. The shame was a low, constant burn, the furnace that refined his character.

The words came to him again, not as a desperate plea, but as a quiet, final statement of fact, echoing the truth he had finally grasped.

"I wish I didn't take it."

He hadn't taken a loan; he hadn't taken a shortcut. He had taken the path to his own undoing. And in the silent, humbling failure of his life, he finally understood the true cost of the transaction: the loss of himself.

Chapter 7: The Lingering Echo

A year and a half passed. The suburban house, its bond finally settled by the bank, was sold to a young, oblivious couple who immediately hired a landscaper to rip out the dead, overgrown shrubbery and a cleaner to deal with the persistent, faint earthy odor that lingered in the shed. They installed an alarm system and a pool cover, sealing off the last physical remnants of Thabo's nightmare. For them, it was a beautiful, fresh start.

But back in the *kasi*, the story of Dr. Mthembu was a slow-fading, persistent lesson, not a spectacular ruin. **Nomusa**, settled back in the small house that had always been the honest foundation of his life, raised her children with a quiet, fierce dedication to frugality and hard work. Her neighbors, who had once seen her husband as a demigod, now saw her as a survivor who had weathered the storm of excessive ambition. The story of the successful doctor who lost everything chasing a suburban mirage became a whispered caution to ambitious young people: *Don't let the new life swallow the old one.*

Zandile, free from the crushing pretense of high-end suburban living, used her sharp, pragmatic nature to start a successful modest business selling handcrafted goods to tourists. She carried the pain of the betrayal, but she rebuilt her life on solid ground. **Ayanda** faded away into the wider city, her only memory of Thabo being a stack of unpaid bills and a lingering bitterness toward men who promised wealth and status they couldn't sustain.

As for Thabo, he remained a nameless face among the million laborers of the city. He was promoted from scrubbing floors to working shifts at a bustling commercial depot, loading and unloading boxes onto trucks. He was a ghost in his old world, and nobody knew that the worn, quiet man stacking crates was once the famous Dr. Mthembu, the man who had traded his soul for an empty mansion.

One clear evening, as the sun set, Thabo finished his shift. He caught his reflection in the greasy window of the truck—a man weathered, aged beyond his years, but with a strange, hard-won peace in his eyes. He had nothing left: no wives, no house, no status. But he also had no debt, no secrets, and no shame greater than the one he carried in the quiet of his own mind.

He was finally free of the crushing burden of expectation. He had traded the expensive lie for a cheap, difficult truth, finding a strange, humble redemption in the sheer, honest effort of manual work.

He walked away from the depot, his footsteps echoing softly in the twilight. The weight of the suburbs was gone. All that remained was the quiet, profound weight of what he had done, and the simple, difficult path of living with it.

Chapter 8: The Consultation

Thabo stood on the depot floor, maneuvering a pallet jack loaded with heavy cartons of imported cooking oil. The work was relentless, the noise a constant, deafening mix of engine rumble and shouted instructions, but it anchored him. He liked the sweat, the ache, the feeling that every rand he earned was the result of a direct, honest expenditure of effort.

He had learned to blend, to keep his head down, perfecting the art of being invisible—a man without a history, known only as "T. Mthembu" on the weekly payroll.

One sweltering afternoon, a new truck pulled into the receiving bay, much cleaner and more modern than the others. The driver who emerged was a familiar, unwelcome face: Sipho.

Sipho, still tailored, still smelling of expensive cologne and cigar smoke, looked effortlessly prosperous. He had likely expanded his "logistics and distribution" empire, now incorporating legitimate, high-volume contracts. He was there to oversee the delivery of a large shipment of high-end electronic goods, likely destined for his own network of illicit markets.

Sipho saw Thabo immediately. The wide, cruel smile of recognition that spread across his face was the same smile he wore in the smoky club years ago.

"Well, well, look who the tide washed up," Sipho drawled, loud enough for a few nearby workers to glance over. He approached Thabo, his voice dropping to a conspiratorial, mocking whisper. "The great Doctor Mthembu. From surgeon to stacker. That's a fall, my friend. A dramatic one. Did you finally get rid of the python, or did it eat the last of your dignity?"

Thabo kept his hands steady on the pallet jack, his eyes focused on the loading dock ramp. He felt the cold pressure of shame, but it was distant now, tempered by the long months of grueling, honest work. The old Thabo—the desperate, image-obsessed man—would have crumpled, perhaps even begged. The new Thabo only felt a weary disgust.

"It was a mistake, Sipho," Thabo said, his voice low and toneless. "The transaction was flawed, and I paid the full price. I'm just T. Mthembu here. Focus on your delivery."

Sipho scoffed, leaning in. "Flawed? No, Thabo. You were flawed. You didn't commit. You wanted the rewards of the darkness without giving up the privileges of the light. But never mind that. I saw Nomusa recently. She asked about you. Looking good, actually. Thriving. Seems you were the thing holding her back."

Sipho paused, then his expression shifted slightly, becoming calculating. "Listen, there's a reason I came over. I have a problem, a serious one. A business partner—he's got a persistent cough, been losing weight. The hospital doctors are useless. They want scans, tests, paperwork. I need a quick fix. Anonymously. You're a doctor, Thabo. A good one, suspended license or not. You know the dark things. Just look at him. A quick consultation, discreetly. I'll pay you well. Cash. Enough to make this job look like pocket change."

Sipho pulled out a thick wad of high-denomination notes and fanned them under Thabo's nose.

The familiar, intoxicating scent of fast, easy money hit Thabo hard. For a dizzying instant, the ghost of the suburban house, the three wives, and the black German car flickered in his vision. He could help Nomusa's family. He could buy a small room, stop sharing a wall with strangers. He could use his *real* skill again.

He looked at the cash, then at Sipho's expectant, predatory eyes, and finally, down at his own calloused, rough hands gripping the handle of the pallet jack. These hands, rough as they were, were clean. They had scrubbed floors and stacked boxes, but they had not harmed a soul or stolen a life.

He pushed the pallet jack forward, rolling it past Sipho's polished shoes and the tempting stack of cash.

"I'm not a doctor, Sipho," Thabo said, not looking back. "I'm a loader at a distribution depot. I don't treat coughs, and I don't take shortcuts anymore. You'll have to use the hospital, or go back to your *nyanga*."

Sipho yelled a curse behind him, furious and incredulous, the crisp banknotes fluttering in his hand. But Thabo didn't flinch. He continued pushing the heavy load, the sound of the wheels on the concrete drowning out the sound of Sipho's rage and the whisper of temptation.

He realized the true, final transaction was complete. The money and the status were irrelevant. He had chosen the difficult, humbling road of truth over the easy, seductive road of the lie. The man who wore the expensive suit was still shackled by his greed. The man in the dusty depot clothes was finally free.

Chapter 9: The Smallest Kindness

A week after Sipho's visit, the depot was buzzing with its usual chaotic energy. Thabo was helping offload a large container when a young man, Sibusiso, a cheerful new recruit, misjudged a stack of heavy boxes. The top row slid, catching Sibusiso's arm and slamming his hand against a steel beam. The noise was muffled, but Sibusiso's gasp was sharp, followed by a raw cry of pain.

Thabo was there instantly. The other loaders froze, unsure what to do. The manager was too far away. Thabo, forgetting the dirty clothes and the disgraced past, simply became the professional. He didn't think; he acted on two decades of instinct.

"Hold still, Sibusiso," he commanded, his voice suddenly clear, authoritative, and utterly focused—the voice of a surgeon in the operating theatre.

He gently assessed the swollen, rapidly bruising hand, checking for capillary refill and testing range of motion. "It's not dislocated, but the radius is likely fractured. We need to stabilize it immediately."

He quickly looked around, his mind already cycling through options for a makeshift splint. He grabbed a thick, clean cardboard shipping tube destined for recycling, carefully cutting it lengthwise with his utility knife. He found a roll of sturdy packing tape.

With a precise, tender touch, Thabo wrapped a clean rag around the injury site, positioned the two halves of the cardboard tube along the forearm, and secured it firmly with the tape, ensuring it was tight enough for support but loose enough to prevent nerve damage. His movements were swift, sure, and elegant—the kind of movements his hands hadn't made in years.

Sibusiso, pale but steadying, looked at Thabo with wide, grateful eyes. "How did you know how to do that, T? You're like... a paramedic."

Thabo tied the hand up in a sling made from a clean piece of canvas tarp. "I used to read a lot of first aid manuals," he replied, the lie coming easily, protective of his new anonymity. "Go to the clinic now. No more work today. And tell the nurse I suspect a mid-shaft fracture."

The foreman arrived, breathless. "What happened? Who did this?"

"An accident," Thabo said, gesturing to the uneven stacking. "I stabilized his arm. He needs X-rays immediately. I'll take him."

The foreman, intimidated by the sudden, competent authority emanating from the simple loader, merely nodded.

Thabo drove Sibusiso to the nearest public clinic, waiting until he was seen before walking back to the depot.

That evening, the foreman approached him, holding out R500. "Sibusiso says you saved his hand. You were fast. I owe you this for showing initiative, T."

Thabo pushed the money back. "Keep it. Just make sure the loading bay is safe tomorrow. That's my payment."

As he walked home, he felt a lightness he hadn't experienced since before the German cars and the three houses. He had used his most valuable gift—not for status, not for money, not for darkness, but for a simple, necessary act of healing. The hands were rough, but the soul was steady. The Doctor was dead, but the Healer was alive, living in the anonymity of a loader. He had found his redemption in the smallest kindness.

Chapter 10: The Scrutiny

The aftermath of Sibusiso's accident brought a subtle, unsettling change to the depot. Thabo had refused the money and returned to his routine, but the silence around him was now thicker, punctuated by glances he couldn't quite decipher. The foreman, a gruff, practical man, was definitely watching him.

One lunchtime, as Thabo ate his small meal alone on an upturned crate, a young loader named Vusi slid onto the crate next to him.

"You're T. Mthembu, right?" Vusi asked, chewing slowly. "Sibusiso is back at work. His arm is set, they say. He's telling everyone you saved him. Said you knew exactly what was wrong, what kind of fracture. That's more than just a first aid manual, man. Are you an ex-cop? Ex-soldier?"

Thabo kept his eyes on his food, stirring the contents of his plastic container. "I just learned from necessity, Vusi. Nothing important."

"Sibusiso said you told the nurse 'mid-shaft fracture,'" Vusi persisted, his curiosity keen. "He asked the nurse what that meant. She was impressed. Said it was exactly right. You don't learn that in a community course, T. You smell like dust and oil now, but you talk like... a professor."

The heat of exposure was stinging Thabo's neck. He offered no reply, simply finishing his meal and walking away. His cover was thin, stretched taut over the massive, forgotten history of Dr. Mthembu. He knew that in a place like the depot, rumors took root quickly and could grow into uncontrollable problems. The last thing he needed was to become a curiosity, or worse, a local target for every ache, pain, and suspicion.

The true test arrived two days later, just before the end of the shift. A delivery truck driver, an older man known as Oom Piet, was climbing down from his rig when he suddenly crumpled, clutching his chest with a look of pure, excruciating agony. He didn't fall; he slid down the side of the cab, his face turning a startling, ashen grey.

Panic erupted. The foreman yelled for someone to call an ambulance. The other loaders gathered around, helpless and frightened, shouting conflicting instructions.

Thabo approached the man slowly. Oom Piet was barely conscious, his breathing shallow and rapid, sweat plastering his thinning hair to his forehead. Thabo knelt, placing his rough, calloused fingers on Oom Piet's wrist. The pulse was weak, thready, and galloping. His diagnosis was immediate and terrifyingly clear: a major myocardial infarction. Every second counted. Waiting for a city ambulance could mean death.

Vusi, the young loader, recognized Thabo's quiet, focused intensity from the Sibusiso incident. "T, what do we do? He's barely breathing!"

Thabo looked at the terrified faces, then down at Oom Piet. This was no fracture; this was life and death, requiring intervention that went far beyond makeshift splints. It demanded the full, terrifying truth of his past identity. If he intervened and failed, he risked full exposure, the ruin of his new, quiet life, and potentially legal repercussions. If he did nothing, a man would die inches from him.

He inhaled, and the dust of the depot tasted like the sterile air of an operating room. The shame of his past was heavy, but the Hippocratic Oath, the one thing he hadn't fully managed to destroy, resonated deep in his chest.

"Move back," Thabo commanded, his voice ringing with the forgotten authority of Dr. Mthembu. "Someone find an aspirin. Ask the manager—*now*—if there's any in the first aid kit. Find two tablets, minimum. And find a blanket, keep him warm, but loosen his collar."

Vusi sprinted off, galvanized by the doctor's tone.

Thabo gently positioned Oom Piet on his side, ensuring his airway was clear. He maintained pressure on the man's sternum with a calm, reassuring touch. When Vusi returned, breathless, clutching two small tablets, Thabo had Oom Piet chew the aspirin, explaining quietly, "It will help thin the blood, slow the clotting."

For the next ten minutes, Thabo was Dr. Mthembu again. He coached Oom Piet's breathing, monitored his pulse, and spoke to him in clear, confident medical terms, utterly focused on stabilizing the man until the ambulance arrived. The other workers, mesmerized by the transformation, stood in silent awe, watching the loader they called "T" fight for a life.

When the paramedics finally arrived, Thabo provided a concise, clinical handover: "Sixty-year-old male, suspected acute MI. Administered 650mg of aspirin, pulse irregular but stable, severe chest pain, radiating to the left arm. Blood pressure is likely plummeting. Get him on nitro and oxygen."

The lead paramedic, startled by the accuracy and the terminology, looked at the dusty laborer. "You're a doctor?"

Thabo stood up, the heat of his action already cooling. He stepped back, wiping his hands on his trousers, returning to the anonymity of the depot floor.

"I'm just T. Mthembu," he said, his voice quiet once more. "I got lucky with a first aid course."

He watched as they loaded Oom Piet into the ambulance. He had saved a life, committing the ultimate exposure risk, but he did it not for status or money, but because he finally had to. The Healer had won, forcing Thabo to face the inevitable: his true identity could no longer be contained by the honest dirt of the distribution depot. The question now was not *if* the past would find him, but *when* it would demand its price for his anonymous grace.

Chapter 11: The Investigation

The next morning, the depot was eerily quiet. The previous day's panic had subsided, leaving behind a nervous tension. Oom Piet was stable, hospitalized, and alive—thanks to T. Mthembu.

Thabo worked his shift, keeping his eyes on the ground, expecting the inevitable summons. It came mid-afternoon. The foreman, Mr. Radebe, a man whose respect Thabo had quietly earned, simply motioned with his head toward the small, glass-walled office.

Thabo walked into the office, the air conditioning feeling arctic on his sweaty skin. Mr. Radebe was sitting behind his desk, not looking at him, but staring intently at a laptop screen.

"Close the door, T. Mthembu," Radebe said, his voice flat.

Radebe finally looked up. His eyes held a mixture of awe and profound, professional distrust. He tapped the screen with a thick finger.

"The ambulance crew, the paramedics, they filed a report. Said the layman on site provided a textbook diagnosis and stabilization. They mentioned the clinical language. Management got wind of it. The insurance company got wind of it. We have liability issues now. They wanted to know who 'T. Mthembu' was, and why he didn't check the 'Doctor' box on his employment form."

Thabo remained silent, watching his reflection in the glass wall.

Radebe pushed the laptop screen toward him. On it was an old news article from a minor online publication. The headline read: **"Prominent Doctor Thabo Mthembu's License Suspended Amidst Ethics Probe."** Beneath it was a slightly blurry photo of a younger, more arrogant Thabo, dressed in an expensive suit, standing next to his now-repossessed German sedan.

Radebe's voice was barely a whisper. "Dr. Thabo Mthembu, the one who lost everything in the suburbs. The one who had three wives. The one who was disgraced. Is that you, T?"

Thabo looked at the image, a lifetime of arrogance and ambition staring back at him. He didn't deny it. "Yes, Mr. Radebe. It is."

"Why are you here? Scrubbing our floors? Stacking our boxes?"

"I needed work. Honest work," Thabo replied simply. "I lost my profession, my life, my reputation. I was given a second chance to live without lies. The money I earn here... it doesn't carry the same weight of debt."

Radebe leaned back, chewing on the end of a pen, weighing the cost and the benefit. "You saved Oom Piet's life. No doubt. If you hadn't, we'd be dealing with a death-in-service claim. But I can't have a disgraced, unlicensed doctor on my payroll. The insurance... the liability... they won't allow it. It's against company policy to knowingly employ someone under investigation by a professional body."

He sighed, pushing a termination letter across the desk. "I have to let you go, T. I'm sorry. The company has to protect itself. But I will give you three things. First, Oom Piet is going to be fine, and he asked for you. Second, I will not mention the *Doctor* part in this termination letter. You can keep your identity."

Radebe paused, then pushed a small, sealed envelope across the desk. "Third, this is two months' severance. For Oom Piet. And for being the best loader I've had in five years."

Thabo picked up the envelope. He had been fired, yet again, but this time, he was not humiliated. He was seen, and his actions had been valued. The loss of the job hurt, but the integrity he had regained was intact.

"Thank you, Mr. Radebe," Thabo said, standing.

Radebe stopped him at the door. "Thabo. That article said 'suspended license.' Not revoked. You are a good man who made terrible choices. Find a way to practice again. The world needs the man who saved Oom Piet, not the man who drove the German car."

Thabo nodded, acknowledging the hard truth. He was again unemployed, forced to leave the only sanctuary he had found. But this time, he wasn't fleeing shame. He was simply moving forward, carrying only the small, heavy burden of his own truth. He walked out, his backpack over his shoulder, the two months' severance feeling like a vast fortune, and the knowledge of his renewed purpose feeling like a map. The road to redemption, he realized, was not just honest work; it was service.

Chapter 12: The Clinic of Dust and Hope

Thabo had been fired again, but this time, the termination was a catalyst, not a collapse. Mr. Radebe's words—*"The world needs the man who saved Oom Piet"*—had given him a quiet permission to exist, and the small severance package gave him two months' grace.

He moved into a tiny, dilapidated room in an old, abandoned industrial area on the edge of the sprawling township. It was cheap, secluded, and free from the judgment of the *kasi* he had disgraced. He spent a week in deep contemplation, the dusty diploma he carried finally seeming less like a mark of failure and more like a tool. His license was suspended, but his knowledge was not. He couldn't practice medicine, but he could serve.

His search for a legitimate outlet led him to the **Bophelo Community Center**, a bustling, underfunded facility deep within the city's most marginalized area. It wasn't a clinic, but a multi-purpose resource center with a small, perpetually overcrowded room designated for basic health services, often staffed by overwhelmed volunteer nurses. The walls were peeling, the air conditioning was broken, and the only advanced equipment was a single, ancient blood pressure cuff.

Thabo walked in, his laborer's clothes instantly blending with the crowd of people waiting for assistance. He found the administrator, a weary, pragmatic woman named Gogo Alice, who looked at the stack of applications on her desk with profound fatigue.

"I'm T. Mthembu," Thabo introduced himself. "I have a lot of medical experience. I'm not a registered practitioner right now, but

I want to volunteer. I can do triage, basic wound dressing, and community health education."

Gogo Alice studied him, her sharp, experienced eyes missing nothing—the slight hesitation in his voice, the roughness of his hands, and the unmistakable air of a man who had been somewhere much higher.

"We need hands, Mr. Mthembu, not degrees," she said bluntly. "And we need commitment, not a passing fancy. If you can clean wounds, organize inventory, and tell a mother when her child needs an ambulance *now*, you are welcome. But no diagnosis, no prescriptions, and absolutely no acting like a doctor. We can't afford the liability."

"I understand," Thabo replied, the humility feeling real and earned. "I only want to help."

He started the next day. The work was immediate, messy, and brutally honest. He spent his mornings cleaning and re-cleaning the small health room, organizing the meager supplies, and managing the queue of patients, ensuring the most critical cases saw the lone nurse first.

He was the perfect triage officer. His medical mind could instantly filter the noise of the symptoms to grasp the underlying threat. He could spot the signs of latent tuberculosis, the early stages of severe dehydration, and the difference between a minor burn and one requiring immediate surgical referral—all without crossing the ethical line. He gave advice that was practical and life-saving: **"Go to the Emergency Room now,"** or **"You must drink two liters of clean water, starting now."**

He began running small, informal workshops under Gogo Alice's supervision—simple health talks in the main hall, standing in front of a whiteboard scarred with old marker residue.

"Today," he would announce, his voice steady, "we talk about **High Blood Pressure.**"

He spoke not as the Dr. Mthembu who drove a German sedan, but as T. Mthembu, the community helper. He used simple analogies, translating complex pathology into accessible, actionable advice.

He taught them how to read the labels on food, the importance of walking, and the necessity of taking their medication *every day*, not just when they felt sick. He didn't preach; he shared knowledge, his medical expertise stripped of its arrogance, now serving purely as a vessel for communication and care.

One afternoon, a young mother, Nomvula, brought in her daughter, who was suffering from a high fever and severe vomiting. The volunteer nurse was out on a home visit. Gogo Alice looked terrified.

Thabo took the little girl's hand. He felt the rapid, weak pulse. He observed the sunken eyes and dry lips. He knew the child was plunging into septic shock, likely from a severe infection, and was minutes from collapse.

"This is beyond us, Nomvula," Thabo said, his voice calm but urgent. "The nearest hospital is an hour away. We need an IV drip *now*. I am not permitted to do this, but if we wait, she will die."

Gogo Alice stared at him, her face ashen. "We can't, T. We have no authority. We have no staff."

"We have life and death," Thabo countered, his eyes blazing with the fierce focus of a man who had lost his soul once and would not lose another on his watch. He had the knowledge, and the center had a small emergency kit, including saline and needles, locked away for the nurses.

Gogo Alice, seeing the child's deteriorating state and Thabo's absolute conviction, wordlessly handed him the key.

Thabo worked with the speed and precision of his old life. He found the vein, inserted the cannula, and started the saline drip. He monitored the child's vitals with practiced ease. Within minutes, the little girl's color began to return, the shock retreating inch by agonizing inch.

When the nurse returned, she immediately called an ambulance, praising Thabo's quick, unauthorized action.

Gogo Alice stood by Thabo as the ambulance sped away. She didn't look angry; she looked profoundly relieved. "You saved that girl's life, Thabo," she said, using his full name for the first time.

"I only started the process, Gogo Alice," he corrected her, wiping the sweat from his brow.

"You crossed the line, T. You know that. You risked everything you have left for a child you don't know. The disgraced doctor... you are a healer, Thabo Mthembu. We can't pay you, and I can't guarantee your protection. But we need you here."

Thabo looked at the scarred whiteboard, the room full of waiting, hopeful faces, and the simple, profound honesty of the service. He hadn't just saved a life; he had redeemed a piece of his own. The dusty community center, not the gleaming hospital, was where his true work lay. He was home.

Chapter 13: The Return of the Past

The success of Nomvula's daughter—discharged three days later, healthy and whole—did what Thabo had spent two years trying to prevent: it made him visible. The story of the "Community Helper" who saved the little girl from the shock spread like wildfire through the marginalized neighborhood. Suddenly, the Bophelo Center wasn't just busy; it was inundated. People lined up not just for wound dressing or blood pressure checks, but for T. Mthembu's 'special knowledge.'

"My knee aches, T. They say you know what to do without the big hospital machines," an elderly man insisted one morning, trying to bypass the queue.

Thabo patiently redirected him. "I can organize your paperwork, sir. The nurse will see you. I am not a doctor."

But the fine line Thabo walked was snapping. The official problem arrived two weeks later, ushered in by the broken air conditioning and the general air of decay. A gleaming black official sedan, the kind Thabo himself used to drive, pulled up outside the center. From it emerged a woman in a crisp, expensive suit, radiating the sterile authority of the city's elite medical establishment. It was **Dr. Molefe**, Thabo's former mentor and the Chief Medical Officer who had signed his termination papers.

She found Thabo in the health room, meticulously counting gauze. He was wearing an old, clean polo shirt, his hair close-cropped, his hands rough but steady. He looked up, and for the first time in years, felt the full, cold weight of his past life's failure.

"Thabo Mthembu," Dr. Molefe stated, her voice sharp and low, carrying a lifetime of professional disappointment. "I should have known. The report from the regional hospital about the child's stabilization was precise. *Too* precise for an unlicensed volunteer."

Thabo straightened up, his humility now mixed with a defensive dignity. "The child was dying, Dr. Molefe. Time was the critical factor. I acted to save her life."

"You acted *illegally*," she countered, producing a folder. "The Health Council takes a dim view of suspended practitioners engaging in invasive procedures, regardless of the outcome. We received an anonymous tip, citing unauthorized practice. I am here to conduct an informal investigation for the Council. I need to know the full extent of your activities here."

Before Thabo could respond, Gogo Alice stepped into the room. She was wearing her usual simple cotton dress, her demeanor quiet but fiercely protective.

"Dr. Molefe," Gogo Alice said, her voice gravelly with decades of fighting for her community. "I am the administrator here. I gave him the key. The full extent of his activities here is helping us survive."

Molefe regarded the older woman with cool professional detachment. "Gogo Alice, I respect the work of this center. But I represent the law. Mr. Mthembu is suspended. He saved a child's life by performing an unauthorized IV insertion—a procedure that falls outside the bounds of his legal status."

"And what does the law say about the standard of care available to this community?" Gogo Alice challenged, stepping closer. "The law requires a child with septic shock to be treated within minutes, not hours. Our nurse was on a house call for a man who could not walk. Our nearest hospital is an hour away by public transport, and the ambulance takes another hour to reach this area. My facility, funded by the kindness of strangers, has one blood pressure cuff and one volunteer nurse spread thin over 50,000 people."

She gestured toward Thabo. "The law suspended *him* for chasing a lifestyle, yes. But his knowledge, his training—that is what this community needed when the law failed it. He crossed the line because the other side was death. He didn't charge a cent. He only asked for a broom and a chance to teach."

Dr. Molefe remained impassive, but Thabo saw a flicker of the old mentor in her eyes, a woman who had once fought for better healthcare access herself.

"I have to report this, Thabo," Molefe concluded, her voice softening slightly. "The breach of conduct is clear. But I will also report the conditions I found here, and the outcome. I cannot protect you from the legal fallout, but I can ask the Council why they prioritize punishing a suspended doctor's unauthorized good deed over funding basic medical care where it is needed most."

She placed the folder back under her arm. "The Council will send an official order, perhaps a cease and desist. Be ready. But thank you, T. Mthembu, for saving that girl. You have finally found a way to use your degree that matters."

As Dr. Molefe's black sedan pulled away, Thabo felt a quiet certainty. The old life had returned, not to shame him, but to validate his new path. He was no longer running from the law; he was standing his ground, knowing that his service, however precarious, was a moral necessity. He looked at Gogo Alice.

"What do we do now?" he asked.

"We wait," Gogo Alice replied, her expression resolute. "And in the meantime, T. Mthembu, you have a queue of thirty people who need their blood pressure checked, and a workshop on basic hygiene to run. Go and serve. Let the law come find us here."

Chapter 14: The Council's Compromise

The official cease and desist order arrived not by fancy sedan, but by registered post two days later—a thick, legalistic document from the Health Professions Council of South Africa (HPCSA). The language was cold, formal, and threatening, citing *Section 54 of the Act*, detailing the penalties for unauthorized practice by a suspended member.

Thabo and Gogo Alice kept the letter locked in the safe, running their small operation exactly as before. The confrontation, they knew, would not be avoided by silence.

It arrived a week later in the form of Mr. Ndlovu, a young, impeccably dressed HPCSA legal compliance officer. Ndlovu was thin, serious, and clearly disgusted by the peeling paint and the relentless noise of the nearby taxi rank. He carried a heavy briefcase and a sheaf of stamped papers.

Ndlovu found Thabo running a workshop on preventing dehydration, enthusiastically demonstrating how to mix sugar, salt, and water to create a cheap, effective oral rehydration solution. The room was packed with mothers and elderly residents.

"Mr. Mthembu," Ndlovu announced, his voice slicing through the air like a paper cut, "I am here to ensure immediate compliance with the cease and desist order issued by the Council. You are to cease all activities that leverage medical knowledge, including these unauthorized health lectures and any form of patient triage, effective immediately."

The room went silent. The mothers looked at Thabo, confusion and fear etched on their faces.

Gogo Alice stepped forward, her body small but her presence immense. "These people are learning how to save their children's lives, young man. Are you telling us that the Council would rather have ignorance than education?"

"I am telling you that Mr. Mthembu is suspended due to serious ethical breaches and is not authorized to deliver any medical advice," Ndlovu insisted, opening his briefcase with a sharp click. "He is a liability, not a healer."

Before Thabo could interject, Nomvula, the mother whose daughter he had saved, stood up, clutching her now-healthy child to her hip.

"He is not a liability, sir. He is our safety net," she stated, her voice trembling but clear. "The big hospital sent my child home with a paracetamol and a shrug. Mr. Mthembu saw her sickness. He put the water back into her body when she was dying. He did what the licensed professionals failed to do. If you take him, you are signing the death warrants of the next child who gets sick here."

An elderly man Thabo had helped manage his chronic diabetes added his voice. "He taught me how to walk again, not with pills, but with truth! He monitors my sugar without charging me the fees of the doctors who suspended him. If he's a criminal, then lock up half the city—we're all grateful criminals."

The barrage of testimony was immediate and overwhelming. Ndlovu, who had expected a simple, sterile compliance procedure, was trapped between his legal mandate and the raw, undeniable evidence of community benefit. He looked at the anxious faces, the small child Nomvula held, and the desperate poverty of the facility.

He stepped back, wiping a bead of sweat from his forehead. "I... I will document the community testimonials. But the unauthorized invasive procedure, the IV line, cannot be ignored. The Council must uphold professional standards."

Gogo Alice seized the opening. "Then let the Council issue a standard. Let them give us a license for a volunteer health educator. We don't need Dr. Mthembu the surgeon. We need T. Mthembu the teacher. He doesn't touch the medicine; he touches the minds. Can the HPCSA really prohibit a suspended doctor from teaching basic hygiene and health education in a place where no other medical professional dares to tread?"

Ndlovu stared at the thick, threatening documents in his hand, then at the desperate faces of the community. He knew the media storm that would follow if he enforced a stop to basic health education.

After a long, tense silence, he slowly packed his briefcase. "I am not authorized to negotiate on the suspension," he said, addressing Thabo directly. "But I will file an addendum to the order."

The final document arrived a week later. It was not a revocation of his volunteer status, but an official HPCSA order that formalized the situation. It stipulated that T. Mthembu was **strictly forbidden** from diagnosing, prescribing, or performing any invasive procedures. However, in an unprecedented move, it recognized his limited role: **HPCSA-Recognized Volunteer, Health Education and Triage Specialist,** operating solely under the direct supervision and liability of the Bophelo Center's registered nursing staff (Nurse Zama and Gogo Alice).

It was a deeply restrictive, legally complicated compromise—but it was an allowance. The law had not crushed him; it had recognized the necessity of his service.

Thabo Mthembu, the man who had lost everything, had found a way to use his knowledge within the rigid structure of the law, not as a wealthy doctor of status, but as a humble, essential servant of the people. He was back in the medical world, not in the surgical theater, but in the Clinic of Dust and Hope, where his true redemption lay.

Chapter 15: The New Authority

Thabo's new position as an **HPCSA-Recognized Volunteer** was a strange mix of privilege and restriction. He wore a simple, laminated ID badge, marking him as official—a status that finally pleased Gogo Alice, who hung the HPCSA letter detailing his limited role in a clear plastic sleeve next to the first aid kit. Yet, the badge was a permanent warning: *Do not diagnose. Do not prescribe. Do not touch medicine.*

He focused all his surgical precision and diagnostic intellect into the legal channels: Triage and Education. He developed a color-coded system for sorting patients: Red for Emergency Room *Now*, Yellow for Nurse Zama *Immediately*, and Green for Routine Checkup or Health Education. This system, rigorous and cold, saved Nurse Zama hours and dramatically reduced dangerous delays, ensuring the center ran with a level of efficiency previously unknown.

The true challenge, however, was not in triage, but in adherence. The local regional hospital, recognizing the Bophelo Center's improved process, began sharing data, showing that a significant portion of preventable readmissions—especially for hypertension and chronic respiratory diseases—stemmed from patient non-compliance with complex medication schedules. Patients often misunderstood *when* to take multiple pills, confused by names, dosages, and the varying requirements of food intake.

One afternoon, Thabo was reviewing a stack of empty medicine containers brought in by an elderly woman who had suffered a massive, preventable spike in blood pressure. She was taking her morning pills at night and skipping her midday diuretics because she thought they made her too thirsty.

Thabo was gripped by the familiar, intense frustration of a doctor seeing a solvable problem fail due to communication breakdown. He couldn't change the prescription, nor could he advise on *why* the medications worked—that was diagnosis. But he could change *how* the patient understood the schedule.

He grabbed a handful of small, smooth river stones from the community garden outside—the kind of stones children used for games. He sat down with the woman.

"Mama," he began, placing four stones in a line. "The doctors gave you four pills for your heart. They are good tools. But we will not call them names. We will call them colors."

He used colored markers to draw a simple symbol on each stone corresponding to the colors of her four pills: **Blue for Morning, Green for Lunch, Yellow for Supper**, and **Black for Bedtime.**

He then handed her a small, empty, plastic egg carton. He used a permanent marker to draw a sun on the first cup (Morning), a plate on the second (Lunch), a moon on the third (Supper), and a star on the last (Bedtime).

"When the nurse gives you your medicine next week," Thabo instructed, his voice low and firm, "you sort them by color into your egg carton, matching the stone to the pill. No reading, no confusion. When the sun is high, you take the Blue pill. When the moon is out, you take the Black pill."

The elderly woman's face, initially clouded by confusion, cleared with comprehension. "Like sorting laundry, T. Mthembu. I can do this."

Thabo had created the **Bophelo Compliance System**—a simple, color-coded, visual medication adherence tool that completely bypassed the need for literacy and complex medical knowledge. It was pure *education* and *process optimization*, firmly within the bounds of his HPCSA mandate.

Over the next month, Thabo and the nursing staff distributed hundreds of these simple, home-made kits, teaching patients how to sort their complex cocktails of medication using the visual cues. The results were dramatic. The rate of readmissions at the regional hospital dropped by over 15% for patients linked to the Bophelo Center.

Nurse Zama shook her head in amazement. "Thabo, you are doing more healing now than you ever did at the big hospital. You are not treating the sickness; you are treating the cause of the relapse. You are teaching them how to live."

Thabo looked at his rough, marked hands. He was no longer trading secrets with the darkness or chasing the ghost of status. He was using his entire intellect, his entire medical training, not to elevate himself, but to simplify and stabilize the lives of the people who truly needed him. He had found an authority greater than the one he had lost—the authority of practical, humble, and life-changing service. He was no longer Dr. Mthembu, the disgraced surgeon. He was T. Mthembu, the architect of hope.

Chapter 16: The Data Speaks

The success of the Bophelo Compliance System (BCS) was not just anecdotal; it was measurable. The regional hospital, overloaded and understaffed, was forced to take notice of the dropping readmission rates for chronic conditions linked to the Bophelo Center's catchment area. This wasn't due to a new drug or a highly paid specialist; it was due to a collection of colored stones and egg cartons.

The hospital management invited Gogo Alice and Nurse Zama to present their findings at a monthly review meeting. Gogo Alice insisted that Thabo accompany them, arguing that the *architect* of the system must explain the process.

The meeting was held in the same boardroom Thabo had once frequented—a sterile, climate-controlled space with a gleaming mahogany table. Thabo, dressed in his cleanest, most pressed work clothes, felt the old, familiar anxiety tighten in his chest. He was no longer the disgraced doctor, but he was still a suspended one, walking into the lion's den of his former life.

The room was filled with the senior physicians and administrators who had once been his colleagues and rivals. He saw the new Chief Medical Officer, a stern man who had taken over after Dr. Molefe moved to a governmental post. And sitting beside the CMO, looking prosperous and utterly bored, was **Dr. Van Zyl**, the specialist whose new S-Class had once triggered Thabo's disastrous final descent into debt and dark magic.

Van Zyl caught Thabo's eye, and a slow, pitying sneer spread across his face. Thabo felt the familiar burn of shame, but anchored himself by placing his rough hands on the smooth back of his chair. He was here to present a truth, not a resume.

Gogo Alice began the presentation, detailing the profound need for accessible healthcare education in the community. Then, Thabo took the floor.

He spoke not as a disgraced colleague, but as a systems analyst. He used the hospital's own data, projected onto the screen: a stark graph showing the dramatic 18% reduction in chronic cardiovascular readmissions.

"This decrease," Thabo explained, his voice even and professional, "is not a medical miracle. It is a logistical solution. Patients forget, confuse, and skip medication due to complex schedules and low literacy. We solved the *adherence* problem by bypassing language and literacy, using simple, tangible objects."

He held up a small egg carton kit. "We replaced 'Take two white pills in the morning and one yellow pill with food' with 'Take the blue stone when the sun is out, and the black stone before bed.'"

He finished his explanation, expecting cynical dismissal, but the room was silent. The CMO, the stern man, leaned forward. "Mr. Mthembu, the numbers are undeniable. This is a profound, cost-saving intervention. We can't implement this system hospital-wide without your expertise. Are you available for a consultancy contract?"

The offer hung in the air: a chance to return to the world of mahogany and consulting fees, a vindication of his intellect.

Before Thabo could answer, Dr. Van Zyl finally spoke, his tone dripping with patronizing superiority. "A consultancy? Come now. With all due respect, this is a clever primary care hack, nothing more. We can have an intern write a manual on this. We shouldn't reward a man who lost his license for serious ethical lapses by bringing him back into the system, even as a consultant. It sets a dangerous precedent."

The accusation landed like a punch, intended to send Thabo scrambling back to the shadows. The room stirred uncomfortably.

Thabo met Van Zyl's gaze. The old Thabo would have fought, defended his past, and lost. The new Thabo merely smiled, a genuine, humble smile that acknowledged the truth of the past without letting it define the present.

"Dr. Van Zyl is correct," Thabo stated calmly. "My past professional failures are severe, and the Council's suspension is appropriate. I am not seeking status or reward. I am a volunteer whose mandate is strictly limited to education, process, and triage."

He turned to the CMO. "I cannot accept a consultancy contract that would compromise the trust placed in me by the HPCSA or the community I serve. However, the Bophelo Center needs funding to expand this system, to hire another nurse, and to buy more supplies. If the regional hospital is serious about improving patient outcomes, you can fund the Bophelo Center directly. My expertise comes attached to the center, or it does not come at all."

Thabo had leveraged his humiliation, his suspension, and his success into a shield for his community. He had turned the tables, using the cold, hard logic of cost-saving data to force the powerful hospital to support the desperate center. He was no longer trying to climb out of the *kasi*; he was pulling the *kasi* up with him.

The CMO looked thoughtful. "A grant to the Bophelo Center for the expansion of the BCS. Contingent on sustained readmission rate decrease. We can do that."

Thabo nodded. He had won the battle without firing a shot, securing a lifeline for his true home. As he gathered his papers, he walked past Van Zyl, who sat deflated and speechless. Thabo didn't gloat. He simply walked out of the mahogany room, leaving the ghosts of his ambition behind, and returned to the Clinic of Dust and Hope, where his simple, rough hands had finally found their purpose.

Chapter 17: The Offer of Forgiveness

The grant secured from the regional hospital transformed the Bophelo Center. They replaced the broken air conditioning, hired a second full-time nurse, and, most importantly for Thabo, secured a large, weatherproof storeroom for his "Educational Materials"—the stones and egg cartons.

Thabo was now the Bophelo Center's indispensable, unpaid engine. His focus was entirely on preventative health and systems efficiency. His greatest satisfaction came not from a complex medical victory, but from a small, handwritten note from a patient: "I am walking more, T. Mthembu. My blood pressure is quieter now."

One rainy afternoon, a well-dressed woman stepped out of a private taxi and walked into the center. She was impeccably dressed, carrying a briefcase, and navigated the chaotic environment with the confident air of someone accustomed to boardrooms. It was **Nomusa**, Thabo's first wife.

Thabo hadn't seen her in two years. She looked stronger, calmer, and older—no longer defined by her husband's status, but by her own quiet resilience. The sight of her sent a wave of pain and regret through him, sharper than any debt collector's call.

He was in the middle of teaching a group of young men about the dangers of self-medicating with alcohol. He finished his lesson, excusing himself to approach her.

"Nomusa," he said softly, using her name for the first time in years.

"Thabo," she replied, her voice steady. She didn't look at his hands or his clothes, but directly into his eyes, assessing the man inside. "I heard the rumors. About Oom Piet. About the child. And about the Council's grant."

"They are true," Thabo confirmed. "I am a volunteer here. I lost my license, Nomusa. I lost everything, but I found a way to use the knowledge."

Nomusa nodded, opening her briefcase. She didn't offer a loan or a reproach; she pulled out a thick, legal-looking file stamped with the seal of a prestigious law firm.

"The Council's suspension was for five years, two of which you served while employed at the depot and here. The ethical breach regarding the *isidliso* was judged as a severe lapse, but the criminal fraud charges were dismissed due to lack of proof. Your medical knowledge was never questioned, only your judgment and ethics."

Thabo frowned. "Why are you here, Nomusa?"

"Because I am a mother who watches the news," she said, her voice hardening slightly. "And I saw Dr. Van Zyl trying to discredit you at the hospital meeting. I saw the man who ruined us trying to claw his way back to status. But the man who stood up for this center... that man I recognize."

She placed the file on the scarred table. "I used the last of the savings I took, Thabo—the money I kept for the children's education—to hire a top medical defense lawyer. I told him your story. Not the doctor who bought the car, but the T. Mthembu who saved the little girl and leveraged the hospital for this community."

"The lawyer believes," Nomusa continued, her voice rising with quiet fervor, "that given your proven rehabilitation, your documented service to an underserved community, and the undeniable success of the Compliance System, we can petition the Council for an early review of your suspension. We can argue for a conditional reinstatement, perhaps limited to public health or non-invasive education."

She looked at him, the weight of the past two years in her gaze. "It is not forgiveness, Thabo. You have to earn that every day. But this is the chance to get your name back, not for the status, but for the work. Do you want to try to be a doctor again, or are you content being T. Mthembu, the volunteer?"

The silence in the bustling center was absolute for Thabo. His heart hammered, not with the panic of debt, but with the profound shock of possibility. The path he had taken, the humility he had earned, had unexpectedly led him back to the very door he thought was closed forever.

Chapter 18: The Test of Intention

Thabo stared at the legal file Nomusa had placed on the scarred table. It wasn't the promise of status or wealth that held his gaze, but the possibility of officially using his full knowledge again—of teaching, of systems, of perhaps even being allowed to administer aid in extreme emergencies without risking his freedom.

"It's not about the money, Thabo," Nomusa said, reading his hesitation. "It's about authority. You have earned the right to have your work recognized and protected."

Thabo spent the evening speaking to Gogo Alice. He explained the offer, and the risk: if the HPCSA review failed, they might revoke his newly granted "HPCSA-Recognized Volunteer" status, crippling the Bophelo Center's vital outreach programs.

Gogo Alice listened, quiet and intense. "The risk is real, T. Mthembu. But if we win, the Council must listen to us. You must go. But you must go dressed as you are now, with the story of these stones in your hands."

With Gogo Alice's blessing, Thabo agreed. Nomusa connected him with the medical defense lawyer, Mr. Nkosi, a man who charged hourly rates that made Thabo's old surgeon salary look paltry. Nkosi was brilliant and utterly pragmatic. He dismissed Thabo's personal history entirely, focusing only on the data.

"We are not arguing for forgiveness, Mr. Mthembu," Nkosi briefed him. "We are arguing for public health necessity. The Council is a regulatory body; they respond to liability and cost. Your Bophelo Compliance System reduced hospital readmissions by nearly 20%. That saves the state millions. The ethical lapse was grave, yes, but the redemption is quantifiable. We propose conditional reinstatement: public health, education, and triage only. No scalpel. No private practice. For life."

Three weeks later, Thabo stood before the HPCSA Ethics and Review Board in Pretoria—the same committee that had suspended him two years prior. The room was intimidating, paneled in dark wood, and the faces of the four board members were a mask of professional skepticism. Seated among them, to Thabo's quiet dread, was Dr. Molefe, his former mentor, who looked at him with an expression of complex scrutiny.

Thabo was introduced not as Dr. Mthembu, but as **Mr. T. Mthembu, HPCSA-Recognized Volunteer**.

The chairman, a severe woman with silver hair, began by dissecting his unauthorized IV procedure. "Mr. Mthembu, you understand that your action, though successful, was a direct violation of your suspension, demonstrating poor judgment and a disregard for the law ?"

"Yes, Madam Chair," Thabo replied, his voice strong and clear, rooted in the hard-won clarity of his current life. "I understand the violation. I maintain that in a scenario of imminent death, where licensed resources were an hour away, my professional obligation superseded my regulatory status. I was guilty of practicing without a license, but I was not guilty of negligence or malice."

He then shifted the focus entirely. He didn't speak of his repentance. He spoke of the **Bophelo Compliance System**. He presented the graphs of readmission drops and read excerpts from the community's testimonials, letting the voice of the *kasi* fill the silent, high-ceilinged room. He explained the river stones, the egg cartons, and the color-coding, showing how systems thinking, not surgery, was his new contribution.

Dr. Molefe finally spoke, her tone cool and measured. "Mr. Mthembu, we see your community work. It is commendable. But tell us honestly: If we grant this conditional reinstatement—allowing you to consult on public health and community processes—what prevents the old ambition, the old debt, from resurfacing? What stops you from using this new, fragile authority to chase status again?"

Thabo paused, taking a deep breath. This was the test. "Madam," he said, looking straight at Dr. Molefe, "the ambition I had was destroyed when I lost my first wife, my children, and my profession. The status I chased was an illusion. The man who stands before you today has cleaned septic wounds with his bare hands and taught a group of men how to use salt and sugar to save a child. I have found an authority greater than my license: the trust of people with nothing left to give."

"If I am reinstated," Thabo concluded, "I will only work for the Bophelo Center and similar public health initiatives. I do not want to practice private medicine or surgery. My condition is this: My license must be tied to a contract that limits my work to non-invasive public health and education. If I ever try to cross that line again, I ask the Council to revoke it permanently."

He had willingly imposed his own permanent restriction. He had sacrificed the possibility of ever being a top-tier surgeon again for the sake of integrity and service.

The board thanked him. Thabo gathered his papers, the mahogany table seeming colder and more distant than ever. As he walked out, he did not know if he would be reinstated, but he knew, with a calm certainty, that he had finally passed the true test of his intentions. Now, all he could do was wait.

Chapter 19: The Verdict and the Vow

The waiting was a dry, consuming anxiety. Every time the worn-out telephone rang at the Bophelo Center, Thabo's heart lurched. Three weeks stretched into a month. He continued his work—running workshops, organizing the medicine adherence kits, and keeping the triage system flowing. The work was his anchor; it was the only thing that kept the phantom pressure of the mahogany boardroom off his chest.

One morning, Nurse Zama handed him an envelope. It was thick, heavy, and bore the official, embossed seal of the HPCSA. It had been delivered to the center's physical address.

Thabo walked outside, needing the dusty, sun-baked earth beneath his feet. He found Gogo Alice tending to the small, wilting community garden, the river stones from his adherence kits scattered around the edges like tiny, colorful sentinels.

"It's here, Gogo Alice," Thabo said, his voice barely a whisper.

Gogo Alice stopped gardening, her face serene. "Read it, T. Mthembu. Whatever the letter says, your work here is already done."

Thabo tore open the thick envelope. The document inside was complex and legalistic, but the core decision was in the second paragraph.

The Council acknowledged the unprecedented nature of his application, his demonstrable commitment to rehabilitation, and, crucially, the quantifiable public health benefit of the Bophelo Compliance System (BCS). It was an admission that their punitive actions, while legally necessary, could not override the practical needs of the public.

The verdict: Conditional Reinstatement.

The conditions were harsh and absolute, exactly as Mr. Nkosi had advised and Thabo had proposed:

1. **Scope Restriction:** License granted solely for Public Health, Health Education, and Systems Consultation.
2. **Procedure Ban:** Permanently forbidden from performing any invasive procedures, including surgery, prescription writing, or clinical diagnosis.
3. **Employment Restriction:** Must be affiliated only with non-profit, state-funded, or registered community health initiatives, specifically naming the Bophelo Community Center.
4. **Permanent Waiver:** Any future breach of these conditions would result in immediate, permanent, and irrevocable license revocation.

It wasn't a return to the glory he had lost; it was a permanent ceiling, a commitment to humility stamped onto his entire professional future. But it was a license. He was a doctor again, restricted, bruised, but officially recognized as a healer.

Thabo handed the letter to Gogo Alice. She scanned the page quickly, nodding once when she reached the section detailing the Bophelo Center's mandatory affiliation.

"Well, T. Mthembu," she smiled, a deep, genuine smile that crinkled the corners of her eyes. "It seems the Council has finally learned to listen to the people. And you are officially stuck with us."

The real work began that afternoon. Thabo's first act as a conditionally reinstated doctor was to draft a contract, a legal document dedicating his renewed license, free of charge, to the Bophelo Center for the next five years.

Later that evening, Nomusa arrived, looking anxious. Thabo met her outside.

"It worked, Nomusa," he said, showing her the letter. "I'm reinstated. Conditionally. No private practice. Only public health."

Nomusa's relief was palpable. She didn't hug him or celebrate; she simply sighed, a deep release of tension she had carried for years. "The lawyer said you were convincing. You finally convinced yourself, too, Thabo. The children are proud of you. They asked me to tell you that."

"Thank you, Nomusa," Thabo said, the words heavy with genuine gratitude. "You gave me the way back. You used your savings not to fix my past, but to secure my future. I will never forget that."

He was still Thabo Mthembu, the man who had fallen, but now he was also Dr. T. Mthembu, the community health specialist, the architect of the Bophelo Compliance System. He had traded the promise of a golden future for the solid reality of an honorable present, and the weight of the expectations was finally gone. He was free to serve.

Chapter 20: The Weight of the Badge

The morning Thabo first pinned his new ID badge to his shirt, he felt a strange, dual weight. It wasn't the heavy brass of his old surgical ID, but a simple plastic card, freshly printed and stating clearly: **Dr. T. Mthembu, HPCSA-Conditional License, Public Health Focus.** The weight came from the restrictions it represented—a professional chastity belt forged of humility and necessity.

The initial celebration at the Bophelo Center was subdued, consisting of a communal cup of tea and a stern warning from Gogo Alice. "The Council watched you fall from the highest place, T. Mthembu. Now they watch you climb back up. Every step must be measured."

Thabo's new role was instantly formalized and expanded. He was no longer just the volunteer triage officer; he was the **Director of Community Health Systems**. The grant money secured from the hospital was immediately funneled into expanding the BCS, and Thabo was tasked with managing the rollout.

His first major challenge was training the new staff, including a second nurse and two local community health workers (CHWs). The CHWs, young women named Zinhle and Thembi, were sharp, enthusiastic, and fiercely protective of their neighbors. Thabo had to train them to operate with the same diagnostic discipline he had imposed on himself.

"You are my eyes and ears," Thabo explained during their training session, pointing at a flow chart he'd taped to the wall. "Your job is to gather data and identify risk. You are not to advise on treatment.

You are not to recommend a drug. Your answer is always one of three things: **Go to the Nurse, Go to the Hospital**, or **Do this specific educational action.**"

He found himself constantly pushing back against the temptation to use his full knowledge. A mother would ask, "Doctor, my baby has this rash, is it eczema?" The old Thabo would have diagnosed and prescribed an over-the-counter cream in seconds. The new Thabo would patiently direct her to Nurse Zama, then spend twenty minutes with the mother explaining proper skin hygiene and the difference between topical creams and oral medications.

The community, however, treated the badge as a full return to grace. They called him "Doctor" with reverence, expecting miracles.

One afternoon, Thabo was reviewing supply orders when a panicked older man rushed in, gripping his chest. His face was gray, and he was struggling to breathe.

Thabo's surgical training kicked in instantly. He saw the classic signs: acute myocardial infarction (heart attack). Time was critical. The immediate, professional response was to administer aspirin, nitroglycerin, and call for high-priority transport—procedures that were now *permanently forbidden* to him.

Thabo felt the crushing weight of the restriction. He was standing a foot away from a dying man, holding a license that prohibited him from saving him.

Nurse Zama was attending to a complicated burn victim on the other side of the center. Thabo had to triage, not treat.

"Zinhle, Thembi!" Thabo barked, his voice sharp with professional urgency, pointing at the patient. "Acute cardiac distress, likely MI! Get Nurse Zama now! Tell her: **Chest pain, 8 out of 10, radiating left arm!**"

As the CHWs scrambled, Thabo knelt beside the man. He wasn't allowed to administer medication, but he was allowed to keep the patient calm and stable until the authorized person arrived. He spoke calmly, guiding the man's breathing, placing him in the optimal position, and loosening his clothing.

When Nurse Zama finally arrived, taking the patient's pulse, she didn't waste a second on diagnosis. She looked at Thabo's pale, sweat-streaked face. She already knew the severity.

"T. Mthembu, get the emergency kit. Call the regional hospital and tell them we are transporting a confirmed code-red MI patient via local taxi, ETA 20 minutes! They must prepare!" she commanded. She then turned and quickly administered the necessary life-saving initial medications herself.

As the taxi rushed the man away, Nurse Zama turned to Thabo, who was leaning against the wall, shaking.

"That was close, Doctor," she said, her voice soft.

Thabo looked at his hands, still rough from the physical labor but trembling from the mental restraint. "I couldn't touch him, Zama. I could only watch and direct."

"And that," she said, placing a reassuring hand on his shoulder, "is exactly what the Council requires. You saved him with your mind, Thabo, not your hands. You have mastered the weight of the badge."

He realized then that his conditional license was not a punishment; it was a constant, real-time exercise in humility and purpose. He had been given a new, difficult job: the role of the vital support system, forever standing slightly back from the patient, directing the flow of care, and ensuring the community survived through knowledge, not surgical brilliance.

Chapter 21: The Unsolvable Riddle

Months passed, and the Bophelo Compliance System (BCS) expanded, becoming a model for community health education in the region. Thabo had found a quiet rhythm, mastering the art of the indirect save—using his knowledge to refine the system, train the staff, and direct resources, never touching the patient himself.

One particularly busy Tuesday, a social worker from the regional hospital, Ms. Fikile, visited the center. She was tracking a troubling anomaly: a spike in pediatric complications linked to an anti-retroviral (ARV) medication switch that had occurred six months prior. The ARV was essential for HIV-positive children, but the new formulation was proving difficult for families to manage.

"We've lost three children in the last month, Dr. Mthembu," Ms. Fikile confided, weary desperation in her eyes. "They aren't dying from opportunistic infections; they're dying from non-adherence. The parents say the new liquid tastes awful, and the dosage instructions are too complex—it depends on the child's weight, which changes constantly."

Thabo immediately recognized the pattern: a systemic failure of patient compliance, just like the hypertension cases he had solved with the BCS. But this was infinitely more complex and deadly. The solution couldn't be colored stones; the dosage changed weekly based on a complex formula linked to the child's growth curve.

He reviewed the hospital's patient notes, which Ms. Fikile had brought. The hospital had simply provided the parents with a printed, laminated table: . The table was densely packed with columns: *Child's*

Weight (kg), *Dose (ml)*, and *Frequency*. For families struggling with literacy and the stress of managing a chronic disease, this table was an incomprehensible maze.

Thabo's medical mind, the sharp, analytical instrument that had once excelled in surgery, saw the fatal flaw immediately. The parents were guessing, or sticking to the last known weight, which led to under-dosing, drug resistance, and ultimately, failure to thrive.

"This table is designed for a nurse's station, not a mother's shack," Thabo muttered, tapping the chart. "The hospital is handing out the formula, not the answer."

He felt the familiar surge of intellectual excitement, the pull of a medical puzzle only he seemed positioned to solve. The solution lay in simplifying the **process**.

He sat down with Nurse Zama and the CHWs. "We cannot touch the medicine. We cannot change the prescription. We can only change the information delivery."

Thabo asked Zinhle to borrow a set of scales from the local market. He took an empty, clear plastic water bottle and an old syringe used for non-invasive measuring.

He realized the hospital was treating weight as a static variable. The truth was, most children fell into broad, predictable weight bands for their age. Thabo's plan was to remove the complex table entirely and replace it with three simple, tangible, and color-coded measurement tools.

First, he designed a simple, color-coded measuring tape. He marked three distinct weight bands: **Red (Small)**, **Yellow (Medium)**, and **Green (Large)**. The CHWs could measure the child's height and circumference and instantly place them in a weight band without using a scale or complex math.

Second, he designed three custom dosing stickers, corresponding to the weight bands. Instead of a volume (e.g., 4.7 ml), the sticker simply showed a fill line on the syringe: .

Thabo instructed the CHWs: "When the child comes in, Zinhle uses the tape. If the tape shows **Yellow**, Thembi immediately hands the parent a syringe with the **Yellow** sticker. The parent fills the syringe to the **Yellow** line, no questions asked, no reading necessary."

He was using his physician's knowledge of pharmacology and pediatrics to create an engineering solution, transforming a differential equation into a color-coded line on a syringe.

When Ms. Fikile returned, Thabo presented her with the **BCS Pediatric ARV Adherence Protocol**: the measuring tape and the custom-labeled syringe.

"The hospital's system is correct in principle but impossible in practice," Thabo explained. "This system respects the parent's intelligence while removing the opportunity for error. It simplifies the variable from 15 dosages down to three actionable color bands. We are not prescribing. We are only simplifying the delivery of the prescribed dose."

Ms. Fikile looked at the system—the simplicity, the elegance, the life-saving potential. She knew instantly that this simple, low-tech solution could save hundreds of children.

"Dr. Mthembu," she whispered, deeply moved. "You solved the riddle the entire pediatric team gave up on."

Thabo felt a wash of profound satisfaction, deeper than any surgical victory. He had saved lives, not with a scalpel, but with a simplified system, proving once again that his purpose was in public service, leveraging the entire weight of his mind, while standing miles away from the strict, dangerous line he was forbidden to cross.

Chapter 22: The Public Stage

The success of the BCS Pediatric ARV Adherence Protocol was too significant to ignore. Ms. Fikile, the social worker, took Thabo's color-coded measuring tapes and custom syringes directly to the regional hospital board. Within two months, the hospital formally adopted the protocol for all pediatric ARV dispensing, noting the immediate and steep decline in severe non-adherence cases.

The hospital management, eager to showcase a positive community initiative and secure more government funding, organized a small press conference to announce the program's success. Thabo, as the system's architect, was reluctantly asked to attend and stand alongside the Chief Medical Officer (CMO) and Ms. Fikile.

The event was held in the hospital's sterile, brightly lit main atrium. Thabo stood uncomfortably in his clean, but worn, clothes, his Conditional License badge feeling heavier than usual. He felt like a ghost at his own wake, surrounded by former colleagues—nurses who offered genuine, supportive smiles, and doctors who offered cool, detached nods.

During the presentation, the CMO praised the "innovative partnership between the hospital's pediatric team and the Bophelo Community Center," carefully side-stepping the fact that the solution came from a disgraced, suspended former surgeon.

When it came time for questions, a journalist directed a query to Thabo. "Dr. Mthembu, how does it feel to be back at the forefront of medical innovation after your time away? Did the break give you a new perspective?"

Before Thabo could answer, a familiar, smooth voice interjected. Dr. Van Zyl, who was standing smugly near the back of the crowd, stepped forward.

"Excuse me," Van Zyl said, addressing the journalist with a look of professional concern. "With all due respect, while Mr. Mthembu's contribution to *process* is noted, we must clarify. This is a system of compliance and organizational simplification. It is a brilliant example of *workflow management*, not clinical innovation. The real medical breakthrough was, of course, the new ARV formulation developed by global pharmaceutical research. Mr. Mthembu merely designed a simple, low-tech way for low-literacy patients to follow the complex instructions devised by licensed physicians."

Van Zyl's intent was clear: to minimize Thabo's achievement and protect the status quo of the clinical elite. He was reducing Thabo's intellectual work from life-saving system design to glorified administrative help.

The cameras turned to Thabo. His first instinct was the old, angry one: to unleash his pharmacological knowledge, to detail the complex metabolic pathways the ARV followed, and explain that designing a simple system to ensure therapeutic consistency was, in fact, the most challenging form of medical innovation.

But he caught Nurse Zama's eye. She offered a subtle shake of her head—a reminder of the vow, the restriction, the line he could not cross.

Thabo took a breath and smiled, his gaze settling calmly on Van Zyl.

"Dr. Van Zyl is correct in his professional distinction," Thabo began, his voice calm and steady. "I am not a clinical innovator. I am a systems specialist. My job is to ensure the brilliant work of the licensed physicians reaches the patient without error."

He held up a custom syringe, marked with the color bands. "When a patient dies because they misread a label, that is not a failure of the drug; it is a failure of the delivery system. I was suspended for my ethical failures, and that suspension prevents me from prescribing or diagnosing. It forces me to solve problems from a new perspective: not from the top of the clinical hierarchy, but from the bottom, standing beside the patient's bed."

"This system," Thabo continued, gesturing to the CHWs who were demonstrating the simple measuring tape, "is a bridge built from my knowledge and the community's trust. It respects that a mother's priority is her child's health, not memorizing a complex dosage chart. If that is only 'workflow management,' then I am proud to be the world's best workflow manager. My focus remains in the community, ensuring every life is saved by simplifying the process, allowing the licensed professionals, like Dr. Van Zyl, to focus on the essential clinical work."

The response was devastating in its humility and its unwavering commitment to the patient. It didn't fight Van Zyl's definition; it owned it, transforming "workflow management" into an indispensable, life-saving necessity.

A reporter quickly changed the subject, asking the CMO if the hospital planned to bring Thabo back onto the permanent staff.

The CMO looked at Thabo. "Dr. Mthembu is an affiliated asset to the Bophelo Center. We rely on his unique expertise there."

Thabo nodded. He was not coming back. He had found his true operating theatre: the dust-filled rooms and crowded halls of the community center, where the only currency that mattered was life and trust. He had endured the public stage and confirmed his new identity, forever restricted, forever serving.

Chapter 23: The National Spotlight

The local press conference in the hospital atrium had a ripple effect far beyond the regional health district. The story of the disgraced surgeon who redeemed himself by inventing a color-coded adherence system—a low-tech solution to a high-tech problem—was picked up by a national news agency and, subsequently, by a prominent international health journal.

The Bophelo Community Center, once a site of quiet, desperate labor, became a destination. Delegations from the Department of Health, and later, representatives from a major international NGO specializing in African public health, started arriving. They weren't there for the hospital's CMO; they were there for Dr. T. Mthembu, the systems specialist.

The NGO, the **Global Health Initiative (GHI)**, saw the BCS not just as a local solution, but as a scalable model for medication adherence across the continent, where literacy, complex polypharmacy, and stretched nursing resources were universal obstacles.

Their field operations director, Dr. Lena Hansen, a sharp, Scandinavian epidemiologist, spent two full days observing Thabo's triage and educational workshops. She saw the quiet authority he wielded, the way he translated medical necessity into practical action.

On the second evening, Dr. Hansen sat with Thabo and Gogo Alice in the small office, the whir of the new, grant-funded air conditioning a persistent background hum.

"Dr. Mthembu," Dr. Hansen began, speaking with clipped, careful precision. "GHI wants to fund the national rollout of the BCS. This means reproducing your system, training thousands of community health workers (CHWs) across four countries, and documenting the results."

Thabo felt a profound surge of vindication. This was the scale he had once dreamed of—not just saving one life in surgery, but improving millions through a system.

"The data supports it," Thabo confirmed. "The simplicity is the key. It needs to be replicated perfectly."

"Precisely," Hansen agreed. "And that brings us to the sticking point. To ensure fidelity in training, we need you to lead the initial training of the master trainers. That training must include the clinical rationale—*why* the dosage changes matter, *why* non-adherence leads to resistance and death. You must be able to train the trainers in the medicine behind the process."

Thabo felt the familiar, crushing pressure of his restriction. He was being asked to perform the very function his conditional license strictly forbade: teaching clinical pharmacology and pathogenesis.

"Dr. Hansen," Thabo replied, his gaze unwavering. "My license restricts me permanently from teaching or performing clinical diagnosis or treatment. I cannot, under any circumstances, teach clinical rationale."

Dr. Hansen looked frustrated. "But you are the only one who truly understands the logic behind the design! If you cannot explain the *why*, the trainers will treat it as magic, not medicine, and they will abandon it when the first small challenge arises."

Gogo Alice stepped in, her hand resting firmly on Thabo's shoulder. "Dr. Hansen, T. Mthembu is forbidden from speaking the language of a doctor, but not from saving lives. He simply uses a different tongue."

Thabo, inspired by Gogo Alice's faith, saw the solution. He stood up, grabbing the river stones and the egg carton kits. He didn't need to teach pharmacology; he needed to teach **consequences**.

“You want the clinical rationale?” Thabo challenged, turning to Dr. Hansen.

"I will teach the trainers the *consequences* of the medical logic, using nothing but metaphor, systems, and simple physics."

He spent the next hour demonstrating how he would train the GHI master trainers:

1. **Dosage (ARVs):** Instead of explaining viral load and pharmacokinetics, he used a simple analogy: "The medicine is a wall, and the virus is a flood. If you skip a dose, you are leaving a **hole in the wall**. The virus flows through and grows stronger. This hole is why you die. The dose must be perfect every time."
2. **Hypertension (BCS Stones):** Instead of explaining blood pressure regulation, he used a visual metaphor: "Your heart is a pump, and your blood vessels are pipes. Your pills are the **pressure release valves**. If you skip the yellow valve, the pressure builds until the pipe bursts. That is a stroke. You are taking the stones not to feel better, but to keep the pipes safe."

He trained Dr. Hansen herself using only these metaphors and visual systems, translating complex pathology into simple, actionable truths.

Dr. Hansen watched Thabo with growing astonishment. He had circumvented the restrictions entirely, proving that his expertise was not in the words on the script pad, but in the life-saving knowledge he distilled.

“The solution is Thabo Mthembu’s communication,” Dr. Hansen finally declared. “GHI will partner with the Bophelo Center. We will hire you, not as a physician, but as our **Chief Global Adherence Systems Designer**. Your contract will explicitly state that your role is the development and implementation of training protocols based on non-clinical, metaphor-driven communication.”

Thabo Mthembu, the disgraced doctor, was now being asked to lead a global public health initiative, forever barred from his old profession, but given an infinitely larger operating theatre: the world. He accepted, the weight of his restricted badge finally feeling light and right.

Chapter 24: The Farewell and the First Flight

The contract with the Global Health Initiative (GHI) was finalized swiftly. Thabo was now drawing a respectable salary, enough to send significant support to Nomusa and his children, and to fund the Bophelo Center's operations for years. His first assignment: lead the master trainer program in Nairobi, Kenya, followed by rollouts in two other West African nations.

The day Thabo officially handed over his responsibilities as the Center's systems director was heavy with quiet emotion. He spent the entire morning running a final training session with Nurse Zama, Zinhle, and Thembi, ensuring they could manage the BCS expansion locally without his constant presence.

"The system is a muscle, not a machine," Thabo told them, pointing to the flow chart. "You must keep exercising the communication. Never guess. Always simplify. Always refer to the Nurse."

He presented Gogo Alice with a detailed, 50-page operating manual for the Bophelo Center—a meticulous document covering everything from inventory management to the precise wording for explaining non-adherence using his metaphors.

Gogo Alice took the manual, flipping through the pages of structured processes and visual aids. She looked up at him, her eyes misty.

"You came here a broken man, T. Mthembu," she said, her voice soft. "You thought your only value was in the blood you could cut and the money you could earn. You learned that true value is in the knowledge you share. You are taking our dust and our hope to the world."

"I am only going because of your faith, Gogo Alice," Thabo replied, clasping her hands. "The Center will always be my anchor. My conditional license remains tied to this place."

Later that evening, he drove the long, familiar route to Nomusa's house. He found her sitting on the porch, waiting. The air between them was free of bitterness now, replaced by a quiet respect for the new man he had become.

"A systems designer for the world," Nomusa smiled, shaking her head. "It sounds like something from your old dreams, Thabo, but without the arrogance."

"It is better," Thabo admitted. "It is real work, not chasing ghosts. I am still restricted. I am still forbidden from practicing medicine, but I can use my mind to save millions. It's a cleaner path."

Nomusa stood and handed him a small, worn leather-bound book. It was his old, annotated copy of *Gray's Anatomy*, the notes and diagrams in his handwriting. "Take this. Not to look back at the past, but to remember the depth of your knowledge. They hired your mind, Thabo. Do not forget how brilliant it is, even if it cannot touch a scalpel."

He left the house feeling a profound sense of closure. He was not repairing the marriage, but he had repaired the relationship with the mother of his children and, more importantly, with himself.

The next morning, Thabo found himself standing in the departure hall of Johannesburg International Airport, holding a passport he hadn't used in years. He was dressed in a new, simple GHI uniform, carrying a briefcase full of his adherence kits—the river stones, the egg cartons, the color-coded syringes. .

He looked around at the gleaming floors and the rushing, privileged crowd. Two years ago, he had been trapped here by shame and debt. Now, he was traveling with purpose, restricted by the law, yet internationally recognized for his humble contribution.

As he boarded the plane bound for Nairobi, Thabo looked out the window. The weight of his conditional badge felt comforting—a permanent reminder that his greatest success came not from regaining his status, but from embracing his limitations. The surgeon was gone, but the healer had finally taken flight.

Chapter 26: The Bureaucratic Barrier

Following the successful training in Nairobi, Thabo and Dr. Hansen took the adaptable BCS framework—now known internally as the **Resilience Adherence System (RAS)**—to Dar es Salaam, Tanzania. The initial rollout was marked by the same enthusiasm from the community health workers (CHWs) who eagerly adopted the local bean sorting and cloth knot dosing methods.

The system's immediate success in two distinct cultural and logistical environments proved its global potential. However, scale brought with it the inevitable friction of bureaucracy and commerce.

Three days into the Tanzanian training, the GHI team was ambushed by a delegation from the Ministry of Health, led by Director Mwangi, a man whose tailored suit seemed to reject the humid coastal air. Mwangi was accompanied by a representative from a South African medical supply conglomerate that specialized in blister packs and manufactured dosing aids.

Director Mwangi was polite but firm. "Dr. Hansen, Dr. Mthembu, we appreciate the work. However, this... *system of agriculture* you are implementing is a logistical nightmare for centralized procurement. We have a standing agreement with **Med-Sync Global** to supply standardized, high-quality, plastic dosing boxes and custom-printed pill cards. This is verifiable, traceable, and frankly, more professional than giving our citizens a handful of beans."

The representative from Med-Sync, a slick salesman named Riaan, smiled condescendingly. "Our solution eliminates the risk of using potentially toxic seeds, guarantees uniform tokens, and supports a proper industrial supply chain. Our boxes cost us about four U.S. dollars each, but they are durable."

Thabo felt the familiar heat of injustice. The plastic boxes were a massive, unnecessary cost that would drain the grant money, enrich a foreign supplier, and inevitably fail the moment the supply chain broke down or the plastic degraded in the heat. It was the same toxic pursuit of high-cost, high-status solutions he had once chased.

Dr. Hansen attempted to reason with them, citing the data on the high durability and zero cost of the local, natural materials. "The beauty of the RAS is its resilience," she argued. "It survives when the power is out and the roads are washed away. It's truly sustainable."

Director Mwangi merely shrugged. "Sustainability is secondary to standardization, Doctor. We have a tender to fulfill."

Thabo knew this wasn't about professionalism; it was about kickbacks and the allure of high-tech imports. He realized he couldn't fight them with clinical science or ethics. He had to fight them with their own weapons: **logistics and finance**.

He stepped forward, his new GHI badge prominent on his chest, deliberately addressing Riaan first. "Mr. Riaan, let us talk about the true cost of your professional solution."

Thabo pulled up a spreadsheet on the projector, transforming his systems knowledge into irrefutable data points.

"A single Med-Sync plastic box costs four dollars, as you stated. It is imported. It has a shelf-life of 3 years in this climate before UV degradation renders it unusable. Replacement cost is 100%," Thabo stated, pointing to the line item. "That is a **$400,000 ongoing capital requirement** for a single region over five years."

He then focused on the RAS. "The Resilience Adherence System utilizes locally available, non-toxic seeds and woven baskets. Initial investment is **zero**. Lifespan is indeterminate, limited only by the durability of the local craft, which can be easily and cheaply replaced by the CHW themselves. Furthermore, every locally woven basket purchase supports the village economy, making the patient the primary supplier. We are trading $400,000 in imported plastic for a **$10,000 local economic injection**."

Thabo's voice was measured, devoid of emotional plea. "The Med-Sync solution creates a dependency that will collapse when the NGO funding leaves. The RAS creates local capacity that ensures patient adherence for generations."

He concluded, turning back to Director Mwangi. "Sir, I am not a physician here; I am a systems designer. My job is to minimize logistical failure. Your agreement with Med-Sync introduces massive, preventable financial and logistical risks. You are paying a premium for a system that is demonstrably less resilient and less effective in the long term."

Director Mwangi, faced with irrefutable, cold, hard data presented by a fellow African professional, shifted uncomfortably. The argument was no longer about beans versus plastic; it was about fiscal responsibility and national resilience.

Riaan, the Med-Sync representative, attempted a final, desperate rebuttal, but Thabo simply pointed to the cost-benefit analysis. "The data shows that Med-Sync's system fails the test of sustainability, cost-effectiveness, and local resilience. We recommend immediate termination of the contract."

Dr. Hansen stepped in, sensing the shift in the room. "The GHI's mandate is the most effective use of global health funding. We follow the data."

The Ministry agreed to trial the RAS in two regions immediately, effectively shelving the expensive Med-Sync contract. Thabo had won the battle not with a scalpel or a prescription pad, but with a spreadsheet, saving millions of dollars and securing the future of the simple, life-saving system he had brought out of the dust of the *kasi*. He was now officially a force for change, using his restricted license to dismantle global barriers.

Chapter 27: The Weight of Absence

The success in Dar es Salaam was a turning point. The Global Health Initiative (GHI) secured significant new funding based on the cost-effectiveness data Thabo had presented. The Resilience Adherence System (RAS) was scheduled for immediate deployment across several West African countries. Thabo's passport quickly filled with stamps, and his days were a blur of airports, spreadsheets, and training sessions, translating complex medicine into simple, metaphorical truths.

He was the celebrated, effective professional he had always wanted to be, but now his success felt distant and cold, mediated entirely by his laptop and scheduled calls.

One Tuesday, exhausted after a 14-hour flight from Accra, Thabo arrived back in Johannesburg for a mandatory week of administrative work at the GHI regional headquarters. He drove straight to the Bophelo Center.

The Center was thriving. Nurse Zama had managed the expansion flawlessly. The local CHWs were confident and empowered. Gogo Alice was sitting in the office, meticulously sorting the Center's financial records.

"T. Mthembu," Gogo Alice greeted him, her smile warm but tired. "You are becoming a legend across the continent. But you look like a stranger here now."

Thabo knew she was right. He no longer smelled of dust and antiseptic; he smelled of recycled airplane air and expensive coffee.

He spent the next few days catching up on the Center's local activities and preparing his national impact reports. On Thursday, he drove to Nomusa's house, feeling a need for connection that his professional success couldn't satisfy.

Nomusa opened the door, and the sight of his children—Luyanda, now in high school, and little Zola—filled him with a bittersweet ache. They were happy, well-adjusted, and living a stable life, funded by his system, but largely disconnected from his presence.

He spent an hour with them, helping Luyanda with a geometry problem and reading a book to Zola. The intimacy felt forced, a scheduled performance of fatherhood.

After the children went to bed, Nomusa sat across from him. "You are famous, Thabo. You are doing important work. But you are never here. You are just a signature on a bank transfer and a voice on the phone."

"I am funding their future, Nomusa," Thabo argued gently. "The money is clean. The work is honorable. This is what I have to do."

"It's not enough," Nomusa said, meeting his gaze. "The children have stability now, thanks to you. But they need a father, not a foundation. They need a man who drives them to school, not one who flies them across the continent."

Thabo felt a chilling resonance with his past. He had chased prestige over presence before, and it had cost him everything. Now, in his redemption, he was repeating the pattern, only this time the object of the chase was global public health, not private wealth.

"The GHI needs me, Nomusa. The RAS is saving lives now because I adapted it in Nairobi and fought for it in Dar es Salaam," he pleaded.

"The Bophelo Center needs you, too," she countered. "And so do they." She gestured toward the children's darkened rooms. "The initial fire is out, Thabo. The system is built. The foundation is laid. Now it needs stewardship, not evangelism."

Nomusa's words were a mirror reflecting his deepest fear: that he was substituting the addictive high of global impact for the painstaking intimacy of local responsibility. He had found his purpose in service, but he was losing his way in the pursuit of scale.

"What are you asking, Nomusa?" Thabo finally whispered.

"I am asking you to choose," she said. "The world will always have a new problem for the Chief Global Adherence Systems Designer. But the man who invented the river stone system only has one chance to be present for his children."

Thabo sat in silence, looking at the familiar walls of the house, walls he had almost lost, walls he had worked ceaselessly to protect from afar. He was restricted from clinical practice, but he was free to choose his life. The weight of his conditional license was heavy, but the weight of his children's need was heavier. He knew, deep down, that the greatest test of his redemption wasn't fighting a bureaucrat or solving a logistics puzzle; it was choosing when to stop flying and when to simply stay home.

Chapter 28: The Third Way

Thabo spent the entire night walking the circumference of Nomusa's yard, the question "I am asking you to choose" echoing in his mind. The dilemma felt like a return to his old life: the all-or-nothing pursuit of success. The surgeon was either operating or he was failing; the GHI designer was either flying to Accra or he was sitting idly at home.

But the new Thabo—the systems specialist—knew that binaries were usually false and that the real solution lay in restructuring the flawed system.

He wasn't forced to choose between scale and presence. He was simply traveling too much because the GHI's training model was inefficient, requiring the Chief Systems Designer to personally indoctrinate every new cohort. The solution was to design a system that trained itself.

The next morning, Thabo called Dr. Lena Hansen, the GHI Director, who was still managing the Dar es Salaam rollout.

"Lena," Thabo said, cutting to the chase. "We need to talk about my contract and the structure of the RAS deployment. The current model is unsustainable for scaling, and frankly, it is not efficient."

"I'm sorry, Thabo," Dr. Hansen replied, her voice crackling over the phone. "The data is fantastic. We can't pull back now. We need you on the ground in Liberia next month."

"That is the inefficiency," Thabo countered, his systems analysis mode taking over. "My value is not in being a keynote speaker; it's in design and quality control. Every time I fly to a new country, I spend three days teaching basics that could be done better remotely. We need to transition from an *Evangelist* model to a **Hub-and-Spoke** model."

He laid out his proposal:

1. **Remote Content Delivery:** Thabo would stop traveling for basic training. Instead, he would use GHI funds to develop high-quality, universally accessible video and audio training modules, translating his metaphors into local languages via local trainers (the "Spokes").
2. **The Quality Control Hub:** The Bophelo Center would be formally designated the **GHI Global RAS Quality Control and Training Hub**. Thabo would be based there, focusing his time on refining the system, analyzing field data remotely, and mentoring the regional master trainers via scheduled weekly video conferences.
3. **Strategic Audits:** His travel would be reduced to four *strategic audit missions* per year, where he would spend a maximum of two weeks on the ground, not training, but troubleshooting implementation failures and designing the next generation of the system.

"This model saves GHI 70% of my current travel and logistical expenses, increases the speed of deployment by utilizing local capacity immediately, and institutionalizes quality control in a stable environment," Thabo concluded.

Dr. Hansen was silent for a long moment. She was an epidemiologist, fluent in efficiency and data.

"Thabo, you just designed a better adherence system for the GHI's internal operations," she finally laughed. "It's brilliant. You're right. We need an architect, not a perpetual traveler."

They agreed to the new terms immediately. Thabo's new title became **Chief RAS Architect and Global Auditor**, a role that honored his professional capacity while drastically reducing his time away from home.

Later that afternoon, Thabo drove back to Nomusa's house. He didn't rush his words this time. He simply presented the solution—the data, the new contract, the promise of the four audit trips a year, and the reality of being home every night, rooted at the Bophelo Center.

Nomusa listened carefully, her expression slowly softening from guarded skepticism to understanding.

"You found a way," she said quietly. "You took the challenge and created a better system for the world and for us."

Thabo nodded. "The biggest design flaw was my own schedule, Nomusa. I was substituting scale for substance. The Bophelo Center is the heart of the system. I learned that redemption is not about chasing the biggest stage; it's about honoring the smallest promise."

He finally sat down next to her on the porch, feeling the afternoon sun warm his skin. He placed his new, official GHI ID badge on the table next to the worn copy of *Gray's Anatomy* Nomusa had given him. He was restricted, but he was finally free. The weight of the badge was gone, replaced by the quiet, grounded weight of home.

Chapter 29: The Architect's Grounding

Thabo settled into his new role as Chief RAS Architect and Global Auditor. The Bophelo Center, once a dusty beacon of local hope, was now the functional heart of a multinational public health initiative. GHI funds flowed in, not for luxurious headquarters, but for high-speed internet, recording equipment, and professional production of the Hub-and-Spoke training modules.

Thabo spent his days at a desk in the quiet office he shared with Gogo Alice, his view a far cry from the glittering city hospitals. He directed video scripts, refined the metaphor-driven training guides, and conducted weekly video conferences with master trainers in Tanzania, Liberia, and Ghana.

The local staff adapted quickly. Zinhle, the Community Health Worker, proved a natural on camera, demonstrating the bean-sorting system and the cloth-knot dosing with a confidence that Thabo's stiff delivery could never match. The system had truly become community-owned.

Six months into the new contract, Thabo faced a final, unexpected audit. He was preparing for a remote session with a team in Mozambique when the door creaked open. Standing there was Dr. Lindiwe Dube, the HPCSA representative who had issued his conditional license, accompanied by a stiff-backed junior official.

"Mr. Mthembu," Dr. Dube stated, her expression unreadable. "We are here for a periodic review of your compliance and the status of the Bophelo Center, which is listed as the permanent site of your conditional practice."

This was the ultimate test. Dr. Dube was here not just to check for a breach of the conditional license, but to assess the reality of his international success.

Thabo welcomed them calmly, introducing them to Gogo Alice and the thriving local team. He showed them the data: adherence rates in the *kasi* were holding steady above 95%, dramatically lowering hypertension-related hospital admissions. He then showed them the monitors displaying the live video feed of the master trainer session he was about to lead.

"The Bophelo Center, Doctor," Thabo explained, "is the Global Quality Control Hub for the Resilience Adherence System, deployed across five nations. I analyze implementation data here, and I audit the regional trainers from this chair."

Dr. Dube spent an hour reviewing the meticulous records—the contracts, the video scripts, the remote data logs. She asked complex, probing questions about the system's logic, trying to catch him out on clinical rationale.

"When a patient is experiencing resistance to the ARV, Mr. Mthembu," Dr. Dube queried, "what is your intervention plan?"

Thabo smiled, a genuine, calm smile. "That is a clinical diagnosis, Doctor, which I am not permitted to make. My intervention plan is to confirm, via data analysis, that the adherence system itself has not failed. If adherence is 100%, I flag the patient record and immediately refer them to their licensed physician, ensuring the physician has the most accurate adherence data possible."

He was a firewall, not a frontline. He was restricted, but his restriction was now his greatest strength—it forced him to focus only on the systemic integrity, which was precisely what had been lacking in global health.

Dr. Dube slowly closed her notebook. She looked past Thabo, out the window to where Zinhle was conducting an adherence demonstration with a group of elderly patients, cheerfully sorting beans and discussing their "pressure release valves."

"Mr. Mthembu," Dr. Dube finally said, her voice quiet. "Your conditional license remains in effect. You have fulfilled the terms of your practice and demonstrated an exceptional contribution to public health that falls outside the scope of traditional clinical medicine. The HPCSA will issue a final report acknowledging your sustained compliance."

There was no praise, no revocation of the restriction—only formal, professional confirmation that he had found a way to practice medicine without practicing medicine.

As she turned to leave, Dr. Dube paused. "I must admit, Mr. Mthembu," she said, looking at the complex system radiating from the simple township room. "You have created a legacy more significant than many fully licensed surgeons."

Thabo watched her go, the feeling of victory not a burst of ego, but a deep, steady warmth. He was not a surgeon. He was not a flying global consultant. He was an architect, rooted at home, using his mind to build structures of hope and resilience for the world. He was the man Nomusa needed, the father his children deserved, and the healer the community had always needed. His redemption was complete.

Chapter 30: Epilogue: The Legacy of Restriction

Two Years Later

The Bophelo Community Center never returned to its quiet existence. It was now a bustling, well-funded hub—a living, breathing case study in sustainable public health design. Gogo Alice, looking stronger than ever, managed the finances with a strict, joyous hand, while Nurse Zama oversaw the expansion of clinical services using the robust, clean data provided by the adherence systems.

Thabo, still the Chief RAS Architect, sat at his desk, but his focus was usually out the window. He was no longer staring at dust; he was watching Luyanda, who was now volunteering at the Center after school, tutoring younger children. Nomusa had started a small, successful catering business supplying meals to the Center's training sessions. Their reconciliation was not a dramatic burst of romance, but a steady, functional rebuilding, brick by brick, foundation by foundation.

The Resilience Adherence System (RAS) had fulfilled its promise. Data from across the continent—Mozambique, Kenya, and Ghana—showed consistent, verifiable increases in treatment adherence and corresponding drops in mortality and drug resistance. The system of beans, knots, and metaphors, born out of necessity in a small South African township, was now a global standard for low-literacy health interventions.

Thabo's work had shifted entirely from troubleshooting to creative innovation. He was now designing adherence systems for tuberculosis treatment and maternal health, always anchored in the principles of local resilience and metaphor-driven communication. His mind, once honed for the precise, bloody work of surgery, was now deployed for the precise, delicate work of saving lives through communication flow.

One afternoon, Thabo was reviewing a new training module when Dr. Lindiwe Dube, the HPCSA representative, walked through the door. This time, she wasn't there for an audit.

"Mr. Mthembu," Dr. Dube greeted him, her tone carrying a new warmth. "The Council has received the final, peer-reviewed study on the RAS impact. It is being published in *The Lancet* next month."

"That is good news, Doctor," Thabo replied.

Dr. Dube sat down. "The Council has reviewed your full performance over the past three years. You have met every condition, every audit, and every term of your license. Furthermore, your contribution to life-saving public health practice is undeniable. The Council has voted to officially **revoke the conditional status** of your medical license."

Thabo felt a slow, unfamiliar thrum in his chest. Freedom. He could apply for clinical practice again. He could return to the hospital, to the operating theatre, to the prestige. The ultimate restriction was lifted.

He looked down at the certificate she had placed on his desk, then across the room to Gogo Alice, who was patiently teaching a group of grandmothers how to use the latest pill-sorting basket. He looked out the window at his children, thriving in the light of his presence.

"Thank you, Dr. Dube," Thabo said, his voice steady. He picked up his old, worn conditional HPCSA badge—the one that had felt so heavy two years ago—and placed it gently in his desk drawer. He did not touch the new, clear certificate.

"I appreciate the Council's decision. But I will not be applying for a return to clinical practice. My license is clear, but my calling is here." He gestured around the Bophelo Center. "The operating theatre is small,

Doctor, but the system is global. I am the architect now. This is where I am needed, and this is where I heal."

Dr. Dube simply nodded, a look of profound understanding replacing her former sternness. She realized Thabo Mthembu's redemption was not about what he regained, but what he chose to keep. He had fallen from grace and found his true path only when he was forced to abandon his ego and use his immense knowledge for the simplest, most profound purpose: creating resilience.

Thabo closed his drawer, the old badge hidden away, its lesson learned. He was a doctor, always, but his true, unrestricted practice was the architecture of hope.

Chapter 31: The Architecture of Hope

Six Months After the Revocation

The old office at the Bophelo Center now had a second desk, smaller but equally cluttered. It belonged to Luyanda Mthembu, Thabo and Nomusa's eldest child. Now nineteen, Luyanda had deferred a university acceptance to pursue an internship at the Center, not in medicine, but in **Systems and Logistics**.

Thabo watched him one morning, a deep satisfaction filling the space the old surgical ambitions had once occupied. Luyanda was building a new supply-chain tracker on a simple open-source platform, designing a system to monitor the depletion rates of the local bean stock across the five RAS deployment countries.

"Dad," Luyanda called out, frowning at his screen. "The Ghana region is consistently over-ordering the white kidney beans for the morning dose, but their adherence rates haven't spiked above the average. The system is consuming resources but not delivering better results. Why?"

Thabo leaned over the desk. This was his true operating theatre. "It's not a data problem, son, it's a human one. Tell me what the white bean signifies."

"The morning pill," Luyanda replied.

"And what is the reality in Ghana at dawn, particularly for women who manage the household?"

Luyanda paused, thinking past the spreadsheet. "They are fetching water, starting the fire, preparing the household for the day. It's the busiest time."

"Exactly," Thabo confirmed. "The adherence system is sound, but the *lifestyle system* is hostile to the white bean's time slot. They take the morning dose, but they use too many tokens because they are rushing and double-counting. The system needs to adapt to the friction point. We can't change their lives, but we can change the design."

Thabo and Luyanda spent the next week developing the **"Two-Stage Adherence Confirmation"** module: instead of simply sorting the token into the basket, the patient had to move the token from the sorting basket to a second, smaller, permanent ceramic dish—the "Confirmation Dish"—only *after* the pill was swallowed. This simple two-step process forced a moment of pause and reduced the likelihood of accidental double-dosing of the beans.

Luyanda launched the module remotely, and within a month, the Ghana region's bean usage dropped by 30% while adherence stabilized.

That success cemented Thabo's final professional decision. Having proven the model and trained the trainers, he resigned from his high-paying position as Chief RAS Architect at GHI. He established a small, non-profit academic consulting firm based entirely out of the Bophelo Center: **The Mthembu Systems Institute**.

His new mission was purely educational: to teach the philosophy of systems design for human resilience, free from the dictates of clinical ego or corporate finance. He offered online courses and in-person fellowships at the Center, not to medical students, but to architects, logistical engineers, and social workers—the people who truly designed human environments.

He never wore a white coat again, nor did he ever practice medicine in the traditional sense. His greatest legacy, as Dr. Dube had suggested, was the architecture of hope—a complex, resilient structure built from the rubble of his own catastrophic failure, proving that a restricted life, when approached with humility and insight, can yield a contribution far greater than the sum of its unrestricted parts.

Thabo Mthembu, the renowned surgeon who fell from grace, finally found peace and profound purpose as the teacher of simple, life-saving systems, forever anchored in the dust of the community that had rebuilt him.

Chapter 32: The Enduring System

Five Years On

The Mthembu Systems Institute, operating from the Bophelo Community Center, became a recognized name in development and aid circles, synonymous with the term "**Resilience Architecture.**" They published papers not in medical journals, but in engineering and social science reviews, analyzing the intersection of human behavior and low-resource logistics.

Thabo's courses, initially taught to a handful of local fellows, now attracted global participants who spent weeks in the township, learning how to replace expensive imports with indigenous ingenuity. They studied the history of the BCS—the egg carton, the river stone, the beans, the cloth knot—seeing in its evolution a perfect case study of systems iteration.

Thabo himself remained anchored. He had long ceased to think about the operating theatre, dedicating his focus to teaching and writing. He crystallized his philosophy into three core tenets, which he inscribed on a large wooden plaque hung above his desk, a visual reminder of his journey:

1. **The Friction Point is the Design Point:** A system is only as strong as the moment it conflicts with real life. The true job of the designer is not to enforce compliance, but to remove friction. (Derived from the "rushing morning" problem in Ghana).
2. **Substitution is Superior to Supply:** Never introduce an

imported component if an indigenous, ubiquitous substitute exists. Sustainability is born from zero capital investment. (Derived from the victory over Med-Sync Global).

3. **Metaphor is the Highest Form of Data:** For a system to save a life, the patient must understand the **consequence** of non-adherence, not the clinical rationale. Simple language and powerful imagery translate complex knowledge into actionable truth. (Derived from his use of "the wall" and "the pressure release valve").

Luyanda, having completed his training at the Institute, was now Thabo's lead partner, traveling occasionally to audit new deployments in South America and Southeast Asia. The father and son were building a legacy together, designing systems that scaled the globe while remaining fundamentally rooted in the local community.

One morning, Thabo stood with Gogo Alice outside the Center. A team of engineers from a major European university were touring the RAS operations, taking notes on the ceramic Confirmation Dishes.

"Do you ever think about it, T. Mthembu?" Gogo Alice asked, watching the activity. "The life you left behind?"

Thabo looked at the plaque above his desk through the window. He saw the surgeon, the arrogant man who had sought perfection in the operating room and found disaster in his ambition. He saw the disgraced man who found redemption in the dust. He saw the free man who chose restriction.

"The surgeon believed that if you cut deep enough, you could fix anything," Thabo said, placing his hand on the wooden frame of the door. "But a system is built differently. It requires patience, adaptation, and the knowledge that the smallest, simplest component—like a river stone, or a dried bean, or a single moment of pause—is the one that holds the whole structure together."

His gaze settled on Luyanda, who was patiently explaining the concept of "friction" to the engineers.

"I found my operating theatre, Gogo Alice," Thabo concluded. "It was never in the hospital. It was always here, in the architecture of hope."

Chapter 33: The Test of the Apprentice

Luyanda Mthembu's first independent systems deployment audit took him to a remote region in the Philippines, working with local partners to adapt the Resilience Adherence System (RAS) for a new diabetes management program. The logistical challenges were immense, involving transportation across numerous islands and cultural norms around food storage that clashed directly with the "Substitution is Superior to Supply" tenet.

Two weeks into the deployment, Thabo received an anxious call from Luyanda via satellite link, his young partner sitting on a makeshift dock, the tropical sun harsh overhead.

"Dad, we have a crisis," Luyanda reported, sounding strained. "The local community won't use the designated tokens—rice grains or dried corn kernels. They see them as food, and using them for medication feels like wasting food, which is culturally forbidden. It's creating massive non-compliance. Our **Substitution** failed."

Thabo leaned back in his chair at the Bophelo Center, the sun streaming through the window, contrasting sharply with the chaotic scene Luyanda described. The easy answer, the quick fix, was to tell Luyanda what token to substitute next. But Thabo remembered his own journey—the necessity of hitting the wall before seeing the architecture.

"What have you done, Luyanda?" Thabo asked, deliberately not offering a solution.

"I suggested using small, colorful plastic beads from a local crafts market, a manufactured solution. It's the opposite of our philosophy, but it works, and they accept it."

"And what is the consequence of that choice?"

Luyanda sighed, the sound echoing across the line. "It's costly, it requires a constant supply chain, and it violates the **Substitution** tenet, introducing dependency. It's the Med-Sync mistake, just on a smaller scale."

"Exactly," Thabo agreed. "You solved a human problem with a logistical failure. Now, tell me, what is the *friction point*?"

"The tokens are too close to food, causing cultural friction. The system itself is good; the component is wrong," Luyanda concluded.

"Go back to the **Metaphor** tenet, son. What does the token represent?" Thabo coached gently. "It represents the pill taken, the task completed. It's an abstract confirmation of action. What is universally available, durable, and **not** considered food, but still carries symbolic weight in their culture?"

Luyanda was silent for a full minute, staring out at the water. Thabo allowed the silence to hold, resisting the urge to offer a hint. He knew Luyanda was cycling through the design principles, moving past the quick fix to the resilient core.

"Shells!" Luyanda suddenly exclaimed, his voice bright. "They are abundant on the beach, durable, cost zero, and they are used for decoration, not consumption. We can use small, distinct shells—mussel shells for the morning, clam shells for the evening—to confirm the dosage."

"Is a shell a ubiquitous, indigenous substitute that costs zero capital?" Thabo asked.

"Yes, absolutely," Luyanda affirmed. "It's a perfect zero-cost token."

"Then you have designed your solution, Architect," Thabo said, a genuine smile in his voice. "Remember, your training here was not about memorizing the answers; it was about internalizing the philosophy. The crisis is not the problem; the crisis is the greatest **Design Point**."

As they ended the call, Thabo sat quietly, watching the sun set over the Bophelo Center. He had resisted the urge to perform the surgery, instead guiding the apprentice to heal the system himself. The enduring legacy of his restriction, he realized, was not just the system he created, but the generation of thinkers he was training to maintain and improve it, armed not with scalpels, but with three simple, revolutionary tenets. The architecture of hope was now self-propagating.

Chapter 34: The Propagation of the Architect

The success of the "Shell Token" deployment in the Philippines became the Mthembu Systems Institute's most potent case study, brilliantly illustrating all three of Thabo's core tenets in action. Luyanda returned to the Bophelo Center not just as an apprentice, but as a proven systems architect.

The Institute's reputation transcended the world of NGOs and development aid. They began receiving invitations from unexpected sources: urban planning firms, educational reformers, and corporate logistical entities seeking to apply the principles of Resilience Architecture to complex supply chains and workplace safety.

Six months after Luyanda's return, the Institute received a request that signified their ascent to the global stage. The **World Health Assembly (WHA)**, the decision-making body of the WHO, was preparing a major global resolution on non-communicable disease (NCD) management in low-income settings. They requested that the Mthembu Systems Institute draft the foundational design framework for patient adherence, officially soliciting the **Resilience Adherence System (RAS)** as a potential global standard.

Thabo read the formal letter, the ornate seal of the WHA making his small office feel suddenly historic. This was the pinnacle of professional validation—the world asking for the system he had created in the shed.

Dr. Hansen, still a steadfast advocate from within the GHI, called Thabo immediately. "They want the paper, Thabo. They need the foundational document defining the methodology. This is it—the official ratification of the BCS on a global scale."

"It's a huge undertaking," Thabo replied, a sense of calm accomplishment settling over him. "It requires analyzing five years of data across multiple continents and translating the philosophy into rigorous academic and policy language."

He walked over to Luyanda's desk, where his son was mapping out the next training schedule.

"Luyanda," Thabo said, handing him the WHA correspondence. "You designed the two-step confirmation system. You solved the food-friction problem in Asia. You are the embodiment of the system's resilience."

Luyanda's eyes widened as he read the request. "The WHA? Dad, we have to dedicate everything to this. We need to analyze the cost-benefit data from Dar es Salaam and Nairobi again, the social impact, the long-term sustainability metrics..."

"No, Luyanda," Thabo interrupted gently, placing a hand on his shoulder. "I won't be leading this project. You will. You will draft the foundational WHA document, coordinate the data, and present the findings."

Luyanda was stunned. "But—the pressure, the politics. This is the biggest thing we've ever faced."

Thabo smiled, remembering his own frantic pursuit of prestige. "The crisis is the greatest **Design Point**, son. I am no longer the man who needs to be in the room. My job is done. I designed the initial system; I fixed the flaws; I fought the bureaucracy. Now, my purpose is to ensure the **Propagation** is resilient."

Thabo stepped away, retreating to his corner of the office. His role as the Chief Architect was complete. He had built the structure and trained the next generation. The final test of the system was not its ability to withstand external pressure, but its capacity for self-propagation—its ability to thrive and adapt when the original builder stepped back.

Luyanda took a deep breath, the challenge washing over him. He picked up his pen, looked at the plaque with the three tenets, and began drafting the global policy document that would enshrine the power of the simple shell and the humble bean into international law. Thabo Mthembu, the healer who had lost his scalpel, had successfully trained his replacement, ensuring that the Architecture of Hope would endure and spread, unrestricted by borders or ambition.

Chapter 35: Global Ratification

The drafting process for the World Health Assembly (WHA) document was intense, requiring Luyanda to synthesize the vast, complex data into a concise, irrefutable policy framework. He worked closely with Dr. Hansen at GHI, who provided the necessary political and academic formatting, but the philosophical core—the analysis of friction, substitution, and metaphor—came entirely from Luyanda and the Bophelo Center's field reports.

Thabo, true to his word, only served as a sounding board, reviewing drafts not for content, but for clarity and adherence to the three core tenets. He was mentoring the architect, not performing the architecture.

Six weeks later, Luyanda stood alone in a vast conference hall in Geneva, presenting the **Resilience Adherence System (RAS)** to the delegates of the WHA. He was the youngest presenter by decades, but he spoke with the quiet authority born of real-world success, not academic theory.

He opened his presentation not with a graph, but with a visual comparison. On one screen, he displayed the image of the expensive, imported Med-Sync plastic dosing box (the subject of Chapter 26). On the adjacent screen, he showed the beautiful, locally woven basket containing the simple tokens—beans, river stones, and shells.

"The box," Luyanda stated, pointing to the plastic container, "represents a cost of four U.S. dollars per unit, 100% logistical failure risk, and zero local economic benefit. It is a system built on supply."

"The basket," he continued, pointing to the local solution, "represents zero capital cost, maximum resilience, and a perpetual local economy benefit. It is a system built on **Substitution**."

He used the story of the Philippine Shell Tokens and the Ghanaian two-step confirmation to prove the tenet of **Friction Point as the Design Point**. He concluded with Thabo's core metaphor, explaining how non-adherence was simply leaving a "hole in the wall," a concept that transcended language and medical training.

The delegates, accustomed to presentations filled with complex pharmacology and billion-dollar budgets, were captivated by the stark simplicity and irrefutable data. The cost-benefit analysis proved that the RAS was not merely effective; it was a radical, necessary overhaul of global health spending.

The resolution, recommending the adoption of the RAS design principles for NCD management globally, passed with near-unanimous support. It was a victory for low-cost, local ingenuity, and a stunning, global vindication of Thabo's journey.

Luyanda called his father immediately from the lobby, his voice thick with emotion. "We did it, Dad. They adopted the framework. The BCS is official WHA policy."

Thabo was standing in the Bophelo Center, watching Gogo Alice train a new cohort of CHWs. He felt the same powerful, grounded satisfaction he had felt the day Nomusa accepted his "Third Way."

"No, Luyanda," Thabo corrected gently. "*You* did it. You proved the system is self-propagating. Now come home, Architect. The world needs the next generation of friction removed."

Thabo hung up the phone and walked over to his desk, picking up the plaque with the three tenets. He looked at the inscription, feeling a deep sense of peace. He had spent his life striving for the highest possible level of practice, only to find that the highest level was defined not by his title or his location, but by the resilience of the system he left behind. The disgraced surgeon, restricted to the township, had given the world a tool for hope that would endure, generation after generation, entirely free of his own ego.

Chapter 36: The Final Component

Luyanda's return from Geneva was not marked by a quiet family dinner, but by a spontaneous celebration organized by Gogo Alice and the Community Health Workers. The entire *kasi* turned out. There was singing, dancing, and a massive feast catered by Nomusa herself, whose business had blossomed alongside the Center.

For the community, Luyanda's victory at the World Health Assembly was their victory—a testament that the wisdom born of their necessity was now guiding the world's health policy. They celebrated the simple elegance of the shell and the bean, and the quiet resilience of the Bophelo Center.

Luyanda, no longer the anxious apprentice, spoke to the crowd with confidence, his presentation refined by his experience in Geneva. He made sure to credit the elders, the CHWs, and, most importantly, the patients who had endured and perfected the system.

Thabo watched from the edge of the crowd with Nomusa, holding her hand. He saw the joy, but more importantly, he saw the deep, structural pride in the community. This was the true measure of the system: it didn't just save lives; it restored dignity.

Later that evening, after the last guest had departed and the sounds of distant celebration had faded, Thabo and Nomusa sat on their porch, the township quiet under the deep African sky.

"He is ready," Nomusa said, referring to Luyanda.

"He is the architect now," Thabo agreed. "He no longer solves problems; he designs resilience."

"And you, Thabo," she asked gently. "Is the wall finished?"

Thabo thought of the metaphor that had saved his career and countless lives: the wall against the viral flood. He had rebuilt his own wall meticulously—shuttering the clinic, enduring the scrutiny, fighting the bureaucracy, and finally, choosing presence over prestige.

"The wall is finished, Nomusa," he confirmed. "And the best part is that I didn't finish it with imported concrete or expensive tools. I finished it with the same simple materials I was restricted to. The wall is built of the community, of the principles, and of a choice to stay."

He reached into his pocket and pulled out the new WHA policy framework Luyanda had brought back, the seal and signatures making it a document of global importance. He didn't open it. Instead, he placed it on the small porch table, weighing it down with his old, worn conditional HPCSA badge—the badge that had defined his darkest years and forced his greatest innovation.

"They revoked the restriction, Nomusa," Thabo said, looking at the two objects side-by-side. "I am free to go back. Free to try to be a surgeon again."

Nomusa placed her hand over his, covering both the weighty policy document and the badge. "But you are a doctor here, Thabo. You have already performed the greatest surgery of your life—the one that healed not a single body, but the whole system."

Thabo nodded, finally releasing the ambition that had driven him for decades. His redemption was complete. It wasn't about forgiveness from the HPCSA or global recognition from the WHO; it was about the quiet, earned peace of knowing he had built something that would endure long after he was gone, something that required his whole, flawed, and finally grounded self.

He picked up the badge, the weight of it now feeling completely neutral—a historical artifact, nothing more. He got up, walked inside, and placed the badge in the very back of his filing cabinet, next to his worn copy of *Gray's Anatomy*. He walked back out, leaving the past sealed away.

He sat down next to Nomusa, turning his focus not to the global policy document, but to the stars above the quiet township. The architecture was complete, and the architect was finally home.

Chapter 37: The Quiet Heart

Ten Years Later

The Bophelo Community Center had grown into a regional campus, its footprint encompassing several refurbished buildings, a small, independent solar array, and a dedicated wing for the Mthembu Systems Institute. Thabo now served as Chairman of the Institute, focusing on curriculum design and global strategy, while Luyanda managed daily operations and international deployments.

On a warm Saturday afternoon, Nomusa Mthembu sat in the garden behind their home, weaving a new pattern into a large, sturdy laundry basket. Her catering business had thrived, and she often supplied the Institute's large international training conferences, her indigenous recipes and organizational skills now feeding global thinkers.

She watched her youngest daughter, Zandi, who was home from medical school for the weekend. Zandi was not pursuing surgery or systems design, but primary care obstetrics. She was sitting nearby, patiently tutoring a group of pregnant women from the community, explaining the critical importance of iron supplements.

Zandi held up two small, smooth river stones. "These two stones must go into the basket every morning," she instructed, referring to an adaptation of the original BCS for prenatal vitamins. "If you miss one stone, you have a hole in the wall. The baby needs every brick."

Nomusa smiled, her heart full. The language of resilience was now simply the language of their home.

Thabo emerged from the house, wearing simple shorts and a collared shirt. He was carrying two mugs of tea and his worn copy of *Gray's Anatomy*. He hadn't opened the textbook in years, but he kept it close—a reminder of the immense knowledge he now used to simplify, not complicate, life.

He sat beside Nomusa, handing her a mug.

"Luyanda just secured a major partnership with the University of São Paulo," Thabo mentioned. "RAS will be adapted for Chagas disease management across Brazil."

Nomusa nodded, unsurprised. "Good. The world always needs resilience."

Thabo opened *Gray's Anatomy* to a random page detailing the complex musculature of the arm, tracing a tendon with his finger.

"I still look at this sometimes," he confessed. "And I remember the feeling of the scalpel, the precision, the weight of the moment."

Nomusa stopped weaving and looked at him, her gaze clear and unwavering. "But the precision you found here, Thabo, is greater. The scalpel could only cut, but the bean, the stone, the shell—they connected. They built something that sustains itself."

She picked up the largest basket she was weaving, a magnificent piece of local craftsmanship. It was the perfect vessel—strong, simple, and beautifully adapted to its purpose.

"The greatest architect doesn't build the fastest building," Nomusa concluded, her hands resuming their rhythmic work. "He builds the one that lasts the longest."

Thabo closed the textbook, setting it aside, the weight of its old authority finally gone. He looked at Nomusa, the enduring strength of his wife and partner, and at Zandi, effortlessly weaving the architecture of hope into the next generation. He understood that his most profound contribution to medicine was the simplest one: the quiet, enduring system of the heart he had rebuilt, piece by piece, right here in the dust of the *kasi*.

Chapter 38: The Permanent Endowment

Twelve Years Later

The Mthembu Systems Institute was flourishing, but its sustainability still relied heavily on grant cycles and Luyanda's successful consulting partnerships. Thabo, watching the constant ebb and flow of international aid funding, realized that the final component of his architecture had to be **financial resilience**. A system designed to last generations could not rely on annual applications.

He decided to step down entirely from operational roles, handing the title of Director to Luyanda. Thabo's new, singular mission became the establishment of a permanent, self-sustaining endowment for the Institute.

He utilized the accumulated success of the RAS deployments. He compiled the definitive portfolio, showcasing how the system had saved billions of dollars in procurement and treatment costs across five continents. He focused particularly on the Brazilian Chagas adaptation Luyanda had secured—a complex system of community tracing and adherence that had stabilized a public health crisis using zero-cost, local tokens.

Thabo traveled to New York, returning to the polished glass towers he had once aspired to inhabit, but this time, he wasn't seeking a surgical fellowship or a global health contract. He was seeking capital for pure education.

He met with the heads of several major philanthropic foundations, presenting his case not as a plea for charity, but as an investment in a proven, globally ratified intellectual property. He refused to accept funding contingent on specific, short-term implementation projects.

"The greatest barrier to global health equity is not a lack of funding; it is a lack of **appropriate design thinking**," Thabo explained in one pivotal meeting. "We do not sell a product; we teach a philosophy. The Mthembu Systems Institute is the only place in the world that teaches the WHA-endorsed methodology of Resilience Architecture, rooted in the three tenets of Friction, Substitution, and Metaphor."

His pitch worked because it was simple, logical, and backed by undeniable data. He convinced the largest foundation, The Gates-Sasaki Health Foundation, to establish the **Mthembu Resilience Fund**, an endowment designed to permanently cover the Institute's operational costs and provide full scholarships to all fellows from low- and middle-income countries.

The endowment agreement was signed in a boardroom high above Manhattan, a dizzying height that would have once symbolized his greatest triumph. Now, it just felt far away from the dust of the *kasi*.

Thabo returned home a week later. Nomusa was managing a training kitchen for new catering staff, Gogo Alice was leading an elder women's council, and Luyanda was preparing for his next systems audit in India.

Thabo sat in his office, no longer preparing a curriculum or reviewing a contract. His task was complete. The system was robust; the leadership was trained; the financial future was secure.

He called Luyanda into the room. "The endowment is secured, son. The Institute is financially perpetual. We are free to teach the philosophy without needing to sell the service."

Luyanda, understanding the weight of the achievement, simply nodded, a profound respect in his eyes. The disgraced surgeon, restricted to the dust, had not just rebuilt his family; he had permanently insured the global reach of his intellectual contribution.

Thabo looked out the window at the thriving campus. The final component of the architecture—the permanent financial structure—was in place. He was no longer the architect of a system, but the keeper of a flame. His life's work was complete, self-sustaining, and enduring.

Chapter 39: The Keeper of the Flame

Six Months After the Endowment

The official transition ceremony was held at the Bophelo Community Center. It was a modest affair, eschewing the grandeur of the Manhattan boardroom for the familiar, grounded space where the system was born. Luyanda was formally invested as the Director of the Mthembu Systems Institute, taking his oath not on a legal document, but on the principles of **Resilience Architecture** inscribed on the wooden plaque.

Among the few invited guests was Dr. Lindiwe Dube, the retired former head of the HPCSA audit committee, who now served on the Gates-Sasaki Health Foundation board—the very foundation that had established the endowment.

Dr. Dube was invited to speak last. She stepped up, no longer stern, but carrying the quiet dignity of someone who had witnessed history.

"Many years ago," Dr. Dube began, her voice resonating across the small courtyard, "I came to this place to enforce a restriction on a brilliant but flawed surgeon. I came here to limit Dr. Thabo Mthembu's practice. What I witnessed instead was the birth of a philosophy. Dr. Mthembu did not simply comply with his limitations; he weaponized them. He took the restriction of not being able to practice clinical medicine and used it to create a system that now saves more lives than he ever could have in the operating theatre."

She turned to Luyanda. "Mr. Mthembu, you inherit a legacy built on the ashes of ambition. The highest achievement of your father was not the RAS itself, but the creation of a financial and intellectual architecture designed to survive his own departure. He is no longer the architect of the system; he is the keeper of the flame, the custodian of the knowledge."

Dr. Dube turned back to Thabo, who was standing beside Nomusa. "Thabo Mthembu, you have demonstrated that the highest level of medical practice is not defined by the height of the hospital, but by the depth of the understanding. The Mthembu Resilience Fund is not a gift; it is a permanent investment in the most valuable medical innovation of our time: the ability to simplify the complex."

As the applause subsided, Luyanda formally accepted the role, promising to uphold the three tenets.

Later, as the guests departed, Thabo and Nomusa walked the grounds of the campus. Thabo finally felt the true, enduring peace he had pursued for over two decades. He had lost his career, his status, and his ambition, only to gain a purpose that was both profound and immortal.

"It is finished, Nomusa," Thabo said, looking at the thriving Institute.

"The architecture of hope is perpetual, Thabo," she corrected him. "It never truly finishes, because the world never runs out of friction points. But you, my husband, are finally free. Free of the weight, free of the need to prove yourself."

Thabo took her hand, the sun warm on his face. He was the former surgeon, the former Chief Architect, the keeper of a philosophy born in a simple shed in the *kasi*. His life was no longer about cutting deep to fix a single person, but about teaching the world how to build simple, resilient walls. And that, he knew, was the greatest healing of all.

Chapter 40: The Doctor's Daughter

Fifteen Years Later

Dr. Zandi Mthembu stood in the clean, modern maternity ward of a regional hospital—a facility that had once seemed impossibly distant to the struggling surgeon who was her father. Zandi was a primary care physician, specializing in obstetrics, and she practiced the highest standard of conventional medicine. Yet, her clinical philosophy was shaped entirely by the systems designed in the dust of the *kasi*.

Her patient, a young woman named Puleng, was recovering from a complicated delivery. Zandi was reviewing Puleng's chart, which showed inconsistent adherence to a critical postnatal nutritional regimen.

Instead of prescribing a complex, multi-drug schedule or lecturing Puleng on compliance, Zandi went to the supply cupboard and retrieved a kit. It wasn't the original egg carton and colored beans, but a formalized, commercially available, WHA-endorsed Adherence System kit: a small, sturdy, segmented box designed for low-literacy users, featuring brightly colored, non-toxic polymer tokens.

It was the RAS, refined and professionally manufactured, yet still conceptually identical to the system Thabo Mthembu had invented under duress.

"Puleng," Zandi said gently, sitting beside her. "We are going to make sure your body heals perfectly, and that you have all the energy you need for your baby. This is your system."

Zandi didn't explain the complex chemistry of nutrient absorption. She used the language of the community, the language of **Metaphor** her father had taught her.

"The vitamins are the **fresh cement** you need to patch the wall where the baby left your body. You must put the cement in the wall every day for six weeks, or the wall will crumble over time. This green token is the morning cement; this blue token is the evening cement."

She showed Puleng how to use the tokens, explaining the **Friction Point** not as a memory failure, but as a conflict with reality. "When you are most busy feeding the baby, that is when you forget. The tokens are your pause. Take the token, take the pill, confirm the action."

Puleng looked at the simple, colorful kit and nodded, understanding instantly. It wasn't a doctor telling her what to do; it was a system guiding her.

Later that afternoon, Zandi visited the Mthembu Systems Institute, which was now attracting PhD fellows from MIT and Oxford. She found her father, Thabo, sitting in his old office, reading a manuscript on game theory and logistics, enjoying his retirement from both the operating theatre and the administrative treadmill.

"Puleng is on the system," Zandi reported, leaning against the doorframe. "It works even better when it's clean and manufactured."

Thabo looked up, his face lined but peaceful. "The system is indifferent to the material, Zandi. It only cares about the **principle**. You used the same three tenets I learned when I was restricted to a few pebbles and beans."

"But Dad," Zandi confessed, "sometimes, practicing medicine feels like a fight between the two of you—the surgeon and the architect. I have the surgeon's training, but I have the architect's mind. Is that a contradiction?"

Thabo closed the manuscript and stood, walking to the window.

"The surgeon," he said softly, "sees the body as a machine that must be cut and fixed. He is focused on the catastrophic moment. That is necessary. But the architect sees the body—and the community—as a system that must be *sustained*."

He turned back to his daughter, the doctor of the future.

"I had to lose my scalpel to learn how to build the wall. You, Zandi, get to wield both. You are the final component of the architecture, the true legacy. You are the Mthembu who heals the body *and* the system simultaneously."

Thabo looked around the thriving, self-perpetuating Institute. He had once believed success was found at the height of a glass tower; he realized now it was found in the simplicity of a river stone, and in the enduring peace of a life finally grounded. The weight of his expectations was gone, replaced by the resilience of hope.

Chapter 41: The Architect's Garden

Twenty Years Later

The old metal shed, the birthplace of the Bophelo Compliance System and the crucible of Thabo's redemption, had stood untouched for two decades, a rusty, beloved monument. It was the place where the ego died and the architect was born.

But on a quiet morning, Thabo and Nomusa, now grandparents, stood before it with a small toolkit. The Mthembu Systems Institute was thriving, Zandi was a leading figure in regional obstetrics, and Luyanda was presenting the Resilience Adherence System to the UN General Assembly. The shed's purpose was complete.

"It's time," Nomusa said, tracing a line in the dust on the corrugated iron wall.

"It is," Thabo agreed, picking up a wrench. "The system is perpetual; the physical reminder is no longer needed."

They spent the morning systematically dismantling the shed. As Thabo pulled down the walls, he found the relics of his past: a faded, color-coded egg carton pinned to a strut, a small bag of smooth river stones, and a rusted-out tin can where he had once hidden his illicit notes.

He held the stones, remembering the desperate, brilliant necessity of that time. The stones were worthless, yet they had created a billion-dollar legacy of adherence.

As the last wall came down, sunlight poured onto the concrete slab. Thabo paused, looking at the empty space. It was neither a lab nor a prison; it was simply ground zero for the Architecture of Hope.

Nomusa brought him a small, clay pot containing a young, resilient acacia sapling.

"We don't need the walls anymore, Thabo," she said. "The system is in the hands of the world. Now, we plant the next stage."

Thabo took the sapling, its roots tightly bound, and knelt to plant it in the center of the old concrete slab.

"A system that sustains itself," he whispered, his hands working the soil. "A structure that is resilient to every shock."

When they were finished, Thabo stood back, leaning against Nomusa. The acacia, the tree of the African savanna, would grow where the shed once stood—a symbol of enduring resilience, adaptability, and local self-sufficiency.

"The restriction saved my life, Nomusa," Thabo said, his voice full of peace. "It took away the glory of the surgeon to give me the quiet power of the architect. I lost the right to cut; I gained the wisdom to build."

They stood there for a long time, watching the sunlight play over the small, growing tree. The journey was over, the wall was complete, and the weight of all expectations, external and internal, was finally lifted.

Chapter 42: The Enduring Architecture (Epilogue)

The dismantling of the shed was the final, private chapter of Thabo Mthembu's story. But the legacy of the restriction, the philosophy born from necessity, continued its global, self-propagating life.

Across the world, the Mthembu Resilience Fund ensured the Institute's long-term survival, perpetually funding the next generation of systems thinkers. Fellows from developing nations trained at the Bophelo Center, learning to audit and simplify global health programs. They carried the three tenets—**Friction Point as Design Point, Substitution is Superior to Supply, and Communication via Metaphor**—into their local contexts, applying the principles to challenges far beyond medication adherence.

In rural Vietnam, the tenets were applied to sanitation infrastructure: local ceramic filters (**Substitution**) were used instead of imported plastic pipes, reducing costs and dependence. The daily action of refilling a small water pot (**Metaphor**) confirmed the filter's maintenance, reducing system failure (**Friction Point**).

In the sprawling slums of São Paulo, Luyanda's adaptation for Chagas disease became a template for tracking environmental health risks, using locally carved wooden insects as compliance tokens.

The greatest triumph was the quiet transformation of the global health community itself. The World Health Assembly's adoption of the RAS philosophy had led to a fundamental shift, prioritizing **resilience** and **local capacity** over centralized logistics and expensive technology.

Organizations that had once dismissed the BCS were now mandated to integrate its core design principles.

Thabo Mthembu, the man who had lost his career in pursuit of high-status, high-risk surgery, became the invisible hand guiding global health policy. He spent his final, fulfilled decades as a grandfather, a mentor, and a quiet custodian of the Institute, his hands busy tending the growing acacia tree where the shed once stood.

He never returned to surgery. He never sought an honorary doctorate or a medal. His vindication was complete in the sight of his daughter, Zandi, effortlessly applying the principles in her daily medical rounds, and in his son, Luyanda, standing on the world stage, defining the future of public health.

The story of the disgraced surgeon was complete. It was a story not of failure and limited practice, but of the ultimate, enduring healing—a systemic cure that began with a few river stones and the wisdom to build a strong wall where a fragile one had once failed.

Chapter 43: The First Stone (Coda)

The acacia tree, planted twenty years prior on the concrete slab of the old shed, now provided a wide, dappled canopy over the Mthembu Systems Institute campus. Beneath its shade, a new cohort of international fellows gathered for their orientation. They were engineers from Bangalore, epidemiologists from Lima, and logistics experts from Kyiv—all drawn by the quiet, revolutionary philosophy born in this *kasi*.

Luyanda Mthembu, now the undisputed leader of the Institute, stood before them. His presentation was not on algorithms or budgetary projections, but on a shallow bowl of river water sitting on a small wooden table. Floating in the water were five smooth, gray stones.

"Welcome," Luyanda began, his voice calm, echoing the gentle authority of his father. "You are here to learn the Architecture of Hope. But we do not begin with a building plan; we begin with the smallest possible component."

He picked up one of the river stones, its surface worn smooth by time and flow.

"My father, Dr. Thabo Mthembu, invented a system out of necessity. He was restricted from using complex clinical language, expensive technology, and a centralized supply chain. His solution was simple: he substituted complexity with resilience."

Luyanda then walked the fellows through the history of the system, recounting the first test cases, the egg cartons, the shell tokens, and the political battles won with a simple cost-benefit spreadsheet.

He turned back to the bowl of water. "These stones, floating in this water, represent a concept. The challenge of global health is not a technological gap; it is a **design friction** gap. We build systems that are too brittle, too expensive, and too complicated for the people who need them most."

He took the bowl and poured the water into a larger vessel, leaving the stones dry in the bowl. "Our mission," he stated, "is to teach you how to analyze the water of complex need, and then find the local stone—the **Substitution**—that is so simple, so resilient, and so appropriate, that it survives everything."

As the orientation concluded, Luyanda dismissed the group. But before they could leave, he walked over to a small, enclosed glass case on the wall—the Institute's most sacred relic. Inside lay the original, cracked, conditional HPCSA badge that Thabo had once worn, and next to it, the first river stone he had ever used for the Bophelo Compliance System.

Luyanda tapped the glass. "The story of the disgraced surgeon ends here, in this glass case. His true legacy is not a medal or a revocation of his restrictions. It is the permanent, undeniable proof that the deepest human failure can lead to the most profound, enduring cure."

The fellows stared at the badge and the stone, grasping the weight of the philosophy. They had come seeking innovation; they found instead the wisdom of radical simplicity.

Thabo Mthembu, sitting beneath the acacia tree outside, watched the new cohort emerge, a quiet smile on his face. The flame was not just lit; it was perpetually burning, tended by the hands of the world he had fought so hard, and ultimately, so successfully, to heal.

Chapter 44: Architect's Legacy (The End)

The shadows lengthened beneath the acacia tree. Thabo Mthembu, the architect of resilience, watched the final group of fellows disappear into the evening, their minds newly furnished with the wisdom of the local stone. He reached down and touched the rough bark of the tree, its roots now deep within the concrete slab of his former failure. The weight was gone, the restriction obsolete, the ambition replaced by quiet fulfillment. The man who had sought to be a savior through a scalpel had become a foundation through a philosophy. The system endured; the community flourished; the legacy was secured. The greatest operation of his life was complete.

Dedication

T*o Nomusa,* whose unwavering belief in the power of the local stone provided the first, most resilient pillar of the wall.

To Luyanda and Zandi, who proved that the architect's legacy is defined not by the tools they wield, but by the philosophy they carry into the future.

And to the community of the kasi, for teaching that true resilience is born not from wealth or technology, but from necessity, simplicity, and hope.

Acknowledgements

This book, and the philosophy it details, would not exist without a deep recognition of the friction points that forge true resilience.

First and foremost, thank you to my family: **Nomusa Mthembu**, whose wisdom provided the first, most powerful tool in the architecture, and whose presence grounded a soaring ambition. To my children, **Luyanda Mthembu**, who became the system's finest implementer and custodiana, and **Dr. Zandi Mthembu**, who embodies the perfect synthesis of clinical knowledge and systemic thought.

I owe an immeasurable debt of gratitude to the **Community Health Workers (CHWs)** and the **elders of the *kasi***, particularly **Gogo Alice**, who taught me that the most complex solutions are often the simplest ones, and that true power lies not in technology, but in communication and trust.

To the institutions and individuals who provided the necessary pressure for transformation:

- To the **HPCSA (Health Professions Council of South Africa)** and, specifically, **Dr. Lindiwe Dube**, whose initial restriction was not a punishment, but a profound catalyst for invention.
- To **Dr. Lena Hansen** and the **Global Health Initiative (GHI)**, for having the vision to recognize the universal potential of the Resilience Adherence System (RAS) and for providing the platform for its global expansion.
- To the **Bophelo Community Center**, which remains the living laboratory for this philosophy, proving daily that local capacity is the true path to health equity.
- To the **Gates-Sasaki Health Foundation**, for their commitment to long-term sustainability through the **Mthembu Resilience Fund**, ensuring that this work is

perpetually funded and accessible to all who need it.

Finally, thank you to every patient who embraced the shell, the bean, and the stone. Your adherence is the enduring evidence that the greatest architecture is built not of steel and glass, but of simple, human resolve.

About the Author

Sibongiseni Masengemu is a South African writer and storyteller known for works that explore the intersection of medical ethics, social resilience, and localized innovation.

Masengemu developed a keen interest in the challenges faced by public health systems across the African continent. Their work often draws inspiration from the ingenuity and resourcefulness found within township communities (*the kasi*), arguing that the most enduring solutions are often the simplest and most locally sustained.

"The Weight of Expectations: A Doctor's Fall" is Masengemu's debut novel, chronicling the fictional journey of Dr. Thabo Mthembu. The story serves as a commentary on the pressures of modernization versus the power of accessible, low-cost resilience architecture. Masengemu weaves narrative drama with complex systems thinking, positioning the book as a powerful meditation on failure, redemption, and finding global significance in grounded, local work.

Don't miss out!

Visit the website below and you can sign up to receive emails whenever Sibongiseni Masengemu publishes a new book. There's no charge and no obligation.

https://books2read.com/r/B-A-LADUC-IKSLI

BOOKS 2 READ

Connecting independent readers to independent writers.

www.ingramcontent.com/pod-product-compliance
Lightning Source LLC
LaVergne TN
LVHW022100200926
848481LV00003B/1002
* 9 7 9 8 2 3 2 4 2 5 7 5 3 *